T0343594

THE
Confidence
WORKBOOK

THE CONFIDENCE WORKBOOK

Copyright © Summersdale Publishers Ltd, 2023

All rights reserved.

Inspired by *Stronger Than You Know* by Poppy O'Neill (published 2022). Text by Caroline Roope.

No part of this book may be reproduced by any means, nor transmitted, nor translated into a machine language, without the written permission of the publishers.

Condition of Sale
This book is sold subject to the condition that it shall not, by way of trade or otherwise, be lent, resold, hired out or otherwise circulated in any form of binding or cover other than that in which it is published and without a similar condition including this condition being imposed on the subsequent purchaser.

An Hachette UK Company
www.hachette.co.uk

Vie Books, an imprint of Summersdale Publishers Ltd
Part of Octopus Publishing Group Limited
Carmelite House
50 Victoria Embankment
LONDON
EC4Y 0DZ
UK

www.summersdale.com

Printed and bound in China

ISBN: 978-1-80007-715-7

Substantial discounts on bulk quantities of Summersdale books are available to corporations, professional associations and other organizations. For details contact general enquiries: telephone: +44 (0) 1243 771107 or email: enquiries@summersdale.com.

THE
Confidence
WORKBOOK

Practical Tips and Guided Exercises
to Help Boost Your Confidence

A N N A   B A R N E S

Contents

Disclaimer

This book is not intended as a substitute for the medical advice of a doctor or physician. If you are experiencing problems with your health, it is always best to follow the advice of a medical professional. Neither the author nor the publisher can be held responsible for any loss or claim arising out of the use, or misuse, of the suggestions made herein. If you have any health issues, consult your doctor before undertaking any new forms of exercise.

Introduction

Welcome to *The Confidence Workbook*, a guide to nurturing a new, confident you.

We all have moments of self-doubt. What about the time you weren't sure if you belonged at a new club or if you were fit enough to try out a new gym class? Or the day your lecturer or boss told you to redo a project and you felt like the stupidest person in history? One minute you're riding high and the next you've come crashing down to earth with no idea how to raise yourself up again.

It's not always easy to be confident, particularly if you're prone to critical self-talk or if other people have put you down in the past, but by picking up this book, you've made a positive step towards healthy self-confidence! In return, this book will support you by suggesting a mix of activities, ideas and proven techniques developed by therapists – such as cognitive behaviour therapy (CBT) and mindfulness – to equip you with a renewed sense of self-confidence, enabling you to live your best life.

You alone are enough.
You have nothing to
prove to anybody.

Maya Angelou

What this book will do for you

This book will help you understand the importance of self-confidence, and the effect your confidence level can have on your overall well-being. You'll learn how to boost your confidence, so you'll have more self-assurance the next time you need to step out of your comfort zone. You'll also discover how to use the self-confidence you already have in some areas of your life to remedy your lack of it in others. There is confidence lurking inside everyone – you just need a few pointers and a bit of guidance to help coax it out. The more you understand yourself, the easier this will become, which is why throughout this book you'll also be spending time working on your sense of self-belief and how you view yourself.

You already have the potential to be bold and wave goodbye to self-doubt – you just haven't realized it yet. Creating a self-confident view of yourself and learning how to act with confidence starts with one person – you. You've got this!

How to use this book

This book is for you if...

- **You find it difficult to say no or you're easily influenced.**
- **You can be indecisive.**
- **You get quiet and shy in social situations.**
- **You worry about your body image.**
- **You prefer to stay in your comfort zone.**
- **You avoid anything that's challenging or risky.**
- **You feel scared of messing up and you try to hide it when you do.**
- **You often overthink things.**
- **You change yourself to fit in.**

If this sounds like you – sometimes or most of the time – this book will help. Being confident isn't just about the ability to smash it in situations at work, college or in daily life; it's about creating positive long-term change to your mindset, and this book is here to help you achieve that.

As you read on, you'll find a variety of ideas and tips on building your self-confidence, so you can develop your self-belief and feel better about yourself. This book is all about you, so your first act of self-confidence is to take ownership of the process and work at your own pace. If something doesn't feel like it's useful to you or doesn't resonate with your own circumstances, it's OK to move on to the next section and just concentrate on the specific areas you want to develop.

PART 1
Confidence and you

Confidence really does affect all areas of our lives. It allows us to commit to opportunities that come our way and to tackle new challenges with aplomb. It helps us to be successful in our personal and professional lives, which is crucial for our overall happiness. Research also shows that people who are more confident tend to achieve more academically.

Which begs the question, if confidence is so important to our overall satisfaction levels in life, why don't we do more to cultivate it? The clue may be in what we perceive confidence to be. Most of us spend our lives believing that confidence is something you either have or you don't. Perhaps we've muttered to ourselves at some point, "If only I was more confident, I could try going for that promotion," or "If I had more confidence, I'd have more friends," as though confidence is an entirely separate entity to ourselves. But confidence resides in all of us, all the time – we just need to learn how to activate it. In this section, we'll be exploring what confidence really is (clue – it's something you "do", not "get"!) as well as our experiences with self-confidence and how having it – or not having it – affects our lives.

So what is confidence?

If we were to write a basic definition of confidence, it might look something like this:

Confidence is having the belief that you can do things well.

Sounds simple, doesn't it? But often the reality is not so straightforward. Our beliefs are shaped by our perception of ourselves. So if we're overly critical of ourselves and our abilities, it's harder for our self-belief to shine through.

Think about it – when our confidence is high, we feel like we can achieve anything. We have the courage to believe in ourselves. We have faith in our abilities and the resilience to cope with life's challenges. It sounds like the perfect recipe for a happy and successful life. But all too often we let a lack of confidence – driven by negative thinking – eat away at our ability to be proud of our accomplishments. It clouds our judgement and makes it difficult for us to be resilient when we get knocked off course.

In addition, many of us (wrongly) believe that we can only have confidence when a specific set of circumstances occurs or we've achieved certain goals, such as passing an exam or losing weight. But confidence is an emotional state, which means that sometimes we feel it and sometimes we don't – it isn't always linked to our abilities, as many high-performing professionals who suffer with low confidence would tell you. Over the next few pages, we'll be spending time getting to know ourselves, as well as learning to recognize the difference between high and low self-confidence.

If you're presenting yourself with confidence, you can pull off pretty much anything.

Katy Perry

Getting to know yourself

It sounds silly, but when do you ever stop to think about who you really are? Sometimes life feels like you're running on a never-ending treadmill of things to do, whether that's completing a project, work commitments, hobbies, laundry, making sure you keep up with friends, the joyless task of life admin – you name it, it's on "The List". Sometimes you don't even have time to write an adequate to-do list in the first place! Time for self-reflection is short; let's change that now.

The better you know yourself – your likes, dislikes, what makes you tick, what makes you want to scream – the stronger your self-confidence will be. This is because knowing yourself gives you the opportunity to be secure in your choices, values and beliefs. If you know what these are, you can always give a true representation of yourself, which is crucial for feeling confident in your own skin.

This is a great icebreaker to introduce you to yourself. Just fill in the answers and say hello to you!

My name is...

If my friends described me in three words, they would be...

I couldn't live without...

I could live without...

I get easily annoyed at...

I feel most relaxed when...

I've always wanted to...

I never want to...

Something no one knows about me is...

If I knew I wouldn't fail, I would...

I was able to overcome...

I learned from...

I am proud of...

In ten years' time I'll be...

What high self-confidence looks like

When your self-confidence is high, you trust yourself to face day-to-day challenges successfully and you have faith in what you're capable of. Having high self-confidence is also self-sustaining. This is because high confidence means you're more likely to achieve your goals and be successful – bringing happiness and self-fulfilment to your life. When you're happy, you're more likely to find the energy and motivation to achieve new goals – leading to a further boost to your confidence, and so the cycle continues.

Here are some of the characteristics of high self-confidence:

- **Being kind to yourself**
- **Being open-minded towards new opportunities**
- **Feeling comfortable saying "no"**
- **Owning your mistakes and learning from them**
- **Feeling comfortable asking for help from others**
- **Being willing to admit when you're wrong**
- **Respecting yourself and others**
- **Being assertive and standing up for yourself**
- **Celebrating your achievements and those of others**
- **Standing up for others and doing what you think is right**
- **Respecting your body and caring for it**
- **Trusting in your own judgement**
- **Valuing yourself**
- **Being willing to change your mind**
- **Being optimistic**
- **Being decisive**
- **Being able to laugh at yourself**

What low self-confidence looks like

When you have low self-confidence, you often feel insecure in life, in relationships, at work or college and at home. The anxiety that results from this feeling of insecurity can make it difficult for you to achieve your full potential. Just as high self-confidence sustains itself by drawing on the positives in your life, low self-confidence keeps itself going by feeding off negativity.

Here are the signs to look out for:

- **Worrying what other people think of you**
- **Lacking trust in yourself and your judgements**
- **Making excuses when things go wrong and blaming others**
- **Believing you're incapable of trying new things**
- **Feeling angry or jealous of other people's success**
- **Comparing yourself to others**
- **Disrespecting yourself and others**
- **Needing other people to agree with you**
- **Needing compliments to feel OK**
- **Putting yourself down**
- **Saying "yes" when you want to say "no"**
- **Believing you're not good enough**
- **Seeing feedback as a criticism**
- **Giving up easily when faced with a challenge**
- **Being pessimistic**
- **Being indecisive**

How do you feel right now?

Stop for a moment and tune in to how you're feeling right now. You might like to find somewhere comfortable and quiet, then close your eyes and take a deep breath. Now you're ready to check in with yourself.

Consider these questions – you can write your answers here or just ponder them.

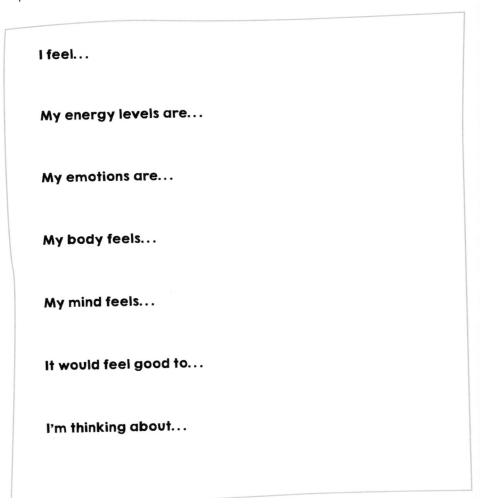

I feel...

My energy levels are...

My emotions are...

My body feels...

My mind feels...

It would feel good to...

I'm thinking about...

What does low self-confidence feel and look like for you?

Think of a time recently when you put yourself down or you worried what other people thought of you. What did that feel like in your mind (and body, if applicable)? How did you react? Write it down below:

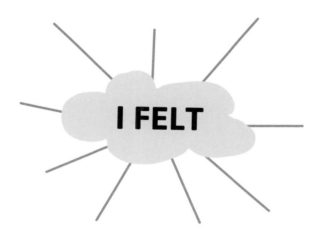

When you've finished, try to think of a time when you felt that your confidence was high. Perhaps you stood up for yourself in a disagreement or you were able to be decisive about something because you trusted in your own judgement.

Thinking about how low and high self-confidence feels for you will help you to identify those feelings in your everyday life. If you can do this, you'll find it easier to modify your mindset when low self-confidence hits.

The self-confidence quiz

Take this quiz to see how high or low your self-confidence is right now. Pick a number for each statement. Choose 1 if it sounds nothing like you and 5 if it sounds just like you. If you're somewhere in between, just go with what feels right.

I feel comfortable speaking in front of people.

1   2   3   4   5

I enjoy the challenge that a new opportunity presents.

1   2   3   4   5

My friends and I encourage each other.

1   2   3   4   5

I feel OK about making a mistake and can admit to it.

1   2   3   4   5

I respect myself, just as I am.

1   2   3   4   5

I feel comfortable offering alternative points of view in a discussion.

1   2   3   4   5

The results

21–30: You have high self-confidence. You're self-assured and you understand the importance of respecting yourself and others. This book will help you understand and strengthen your self-confidence even more, as well as recognize the signs of low self-confidence in others.

11–20: You have average levels of self-confidence but should build it up some more. You know how to give yourself a boost of positivity when you need it – which is great – but there are probably areas in which your self-confidence dips. Strengthening your confidence will help you feel good about yourself, even when you're faced with a challenge.

0–10: Your self-confidence is low. You tend to put other people's feelings and needs in front of your own and prefer to stay in your comfort zone rather than seek out new opportunities. Your feelings do matter, and it's OK to go one step at a time as you regain your confidence – keep reading for activities and advice to build yourself back up.

What affects your self-confidence?

A big part of life is accepting it comes with good times and tough times. While you may not enjoy life very much when times are tough, it is normal and something you share with everyone else on the planet.

But as life goes up and down, so does your confidence. Some circumstances can profoundly affect your sense of self-worth and those are the situations that are likely to lead to low self-confidence. Confidence levels are also driven by what's going on inside your head, particularly your own thoughts and inner voice – and this may or may not have an external trigger.

Confused? Don't panic! We'll be looking at this in more detail later. In the meantime, here are just a few of the things that can affect your self-confidence:

Financial matters

Appearance and body image

Relationships

Age

Education

Work/college

Social media

Past trauma

Upbringing

How low self-confidence can affect your life

Low self-confidence can play into every aspect of your life: just look at the list on the previous page! It affects how you think about yourself, how you react to situations and what actions you take throughout your life.

When you let negative thoughts – either generated by you or via other people – bully their way into your mindset, it undermines the way you feel about yourself. This can have profound consequences for your confidence levels and, as a result, how happy you are in life.

Let's look at an example:

Claire had a happy childhood and was brought up in a supportive family. She performed well at school and college and, as an adult, was able to secure a senior role in her dream company. She was always complimented on how capable she was and felt she could confidently tackle any situation at work or at home.

But after one particularly gruelling work project which had caused Claire, her colleagues and her manager a lot of stress and anxiety, her boss snapped at her, saying, "You're not as clever as you think you are."

This triggered Claire's deep-rooted fear that she wasn't smart enough or good enough to be successful. She began to find it difficult to be assertive at work and stopped expressing her views at team meetings. Over time, she felt less able to cope with the demands of her job and noticed she was being overlooked for new projects. Her worry and anxiety about her lack of success at work made home life difficult too, and her relationships with loved ones suffered as a result.

In Claire's case, a negative belief – that she may not even have been aware she was carrying around in her head – was triggered by the harsh words of her boss. This example may seem exaggerated, but it's useful for exploring the knock-on effect of low self-confidence.

The problem is, once that distrust in yourself has been activated, your whole outlook changes. You start to view everything in life through a filter of negativity. You begin looking for examples that you're not clever enough and, once you've had that negative belief confirmed, it perpetuates low self-confidence.

Can you go from low to high self-confidence?

With a little commitment and patience, you can refocus your mindset so that you're not stuck in a negative loop. Your limiting beliefs won't suddenly disappear, but over time they will lose their grip on your thoughts and actions.

Spend a moment reflecting on what your life would be like if you felt more confident. If you feel comfortable write some notes below.

If I were more confident...

e.g. "I'd find it easier to move on when I make mistakes and learn from them" or "I'd question my own judgement less and make assertive decisions".

_____

_____

_____

_____

_____

_____

Over the next two sections we'll be looking at how to tackle this change in thinking and the steps you can take to boost your confidence levels, such as practising mindfulness and using positive affirmations.

Building confidence comes from overcoming the voice in your head that says you are not capable; silence the noise and then prove it wrong.

Sam Owen

PART 2

Confidence boosters

Self-confidence isn't something you can gain overnight – it's a skill you need to nurture and train over a period of time. After all, you wouldn't wake up one morning and put on your trainers to run a marathon when the furthest you've ever managed before is to the nearest bus stop. Training your brain is no different. How you see yourself and treat yourself defines how others will treat you. Self-confidence is a vital skill because it inspires you to be the best version of yourself, which in turn will inspire others to believe in you.

In this section, we'll be exploring some tips that can boost your self-confidence, which will help you to establish a healthier, more positive mindset.

What makes you feel confident and how can you do more of it?

One of the most amazing things about humans is that we are all utterly unique – no one person is quite like another. This means everyone has different things that makes them feel good and, while we might share the things that make us tick with a group of like-minded individuals, our experience of any one activity will be completely different to theirs. We all enjoy doing things that give us the feel-good factor, so it makes sense that doing *more* of those things will help to boost our confidence in the short term and build it up in the long run.

Let's identify what gives you that feel-good factor. A fantastic way to start this process is to look for patterns in your week. Try taking time out at the end of each day to reflect on when you felt at your most confident.

Briefly describe your day. What were you doing when you were feeling confident? Write as much detail as you can, even the mundane stuff (successfully cooking dinner counts!).

Using your notes, try to identify any patterns. What are you doing on the days that your confidence felt high? What didn't make you feel good?

How could you do more of the things that make you feel good? Can you do one of them every day?

What drains your confidence and how can you do less of it?

Most people have days where everything seems to go wrong. Maybe you trip over running for the bus, then you miss your stop and the journey takes twice as long. Then, because of that mistake, you miss an important appointment. At the end of the day you hobble home to hide under a duvet and pray that nothing else goes wrong. Your confidence in your ability may be in shreds, but you know it's just one of those days and tomorrow will be better.

However, sometimes those feelings of low confidence stick around a bit longer and specific things – people, places, situations – can leave you feeling bad about yourself. Maybe these are obvious, like messing something up at work or spending time with someone who can be overly critical of how you live your life. Often, however, low self-confidence can be triggered by something that seems insignificant, but to you is a sure-fire way of draining your assurance.

Perhaps you dread going on social media, even though you feel compelled to, because one of your friends seems to live the perfect life and yours looks humdrum in comparison. Or you spend longer than is healthy overthinking a throwaway comment your partner made about your new haircut.

If you can identify what drains your confidence, you can practise damage limitation, which will help to banish low confidence from your daily life.

Take a moment to think about what pushes your low self-confidence button. Can you think of two or three situations that are guaranteed to knock your confidence? For example: "Spending too long comparing my life to other people on social media."

Could you change your routine or habits so you spend less time doing these things or find a different way of doing them? For example: "I could set a timer for my daily check-in with social media so I'm only on it for 20 minutes a day. I could unfollow the accounts that I know make me feel insecure."

If not, are there changes you could make that would help you to feel better about yourself? For example: "I can choose not to go on social media when I'm feeling vulnerable."

Affirmations for confidence

An affirmation is a short, positive sentence to help you challenge negative thoughts and feel more confident. Research has shown that repeating positive affirmations on a regular basis can have a powerful impact on your mindset. The theory is that the more you repeat them, the more you believe them.

Choose a different one each morning depending on how you're feeling and spend five to ten minutes saying it to yourself. Affirmations are best said aloud in front of a mirror, but you can think or say them to yourself anytime, anywhere. Different affirmations work for different people, so try these and see which ones are a good fit for you:

- **I have the power to do incredible things.**
- **I'm confident in myself and my abilities.**
- **I can achieve anything I put my mind to.**
- **I trust in the decisions I make.**
- **I'm proud of myself and my achievements.**
- **I live each day feeling confident and grateful.**
- **I can take it one step at a time, and that's OK.**
- **I am strong.**
- **I respect myself.**
- **I can say "no".**
- **My point of view is as valid as everyone else's.**
- **I feel empowered to be the best I can be.**

Use the space below to write your own – then you can personalize them as much as you like depending on what you want to achieve.

Top tip: Write your affirmations on sticky notes and place them where you'll see them every day for maximum positivity.

Talk about your feelings

Sharing how you're feeling with someone close to you can be a positive step towards making changes for the better. Telling someone else that you're struggling with your confidence might feel a little strange or even embarrassing, but research shows that discussing your feelings with a trusted person can have an instant, positive effect on your emotions by reducing anxiety and other negative emotions. This could be because naming our emotions activates the right side of the brain which is responsible for emotional intelligence. This means the effect of the amygdala – the part of our brain that helps us to control both positive and negative emotions – is reduced. Talk to someone you trust and feel comfortable sharing your feelings with. There's a good chance they may not have realized you were unhappy and your confidence was suffering. If they're a truly supportive friend or loved one, they'll be glad you felt able to open up to them and give them the opportunity to help you.

Most importantly, be gentle with yourself and know there are people who want to help.

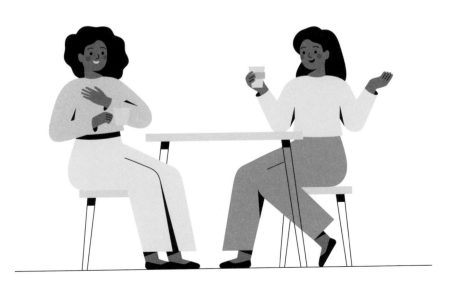

Talking tips

1. If talking face to face feels too much, try writing a letter, email or text to your loved one instead. This is a good way to introduce your problem as it gives them the opportunity to digest the information and reflect on it. You can always follow up with each other in person once you feel comfortable doing so.

2. There are lots of people you can reach out to: family, trusted friends and work colleagues. If you'd feel more comfortable talking to someone who is experiencing the same lack of confidence as you, you could try an online community or forum. You'll be able to post anonymously and gain advice from a group of people who understand what you're going through.

3. When you speak to someone, make it clear whether you would like them just to listen or if you are looking for advice.

See the resources list on pages 155–157 for more ideas about where you can find support.

Who can you talk to?

Who do you turn to when times are tough? Think about the person or people in your life you trust and feel comfortable with. Write their name(s) here. What makes them a good listener?

If you don't have someone like that in your life, skip to page 157 for other places you can turn to for support. But know that you're not alone and help is always available.

Give yourself a pep talk

A pep talk is a positive monologue you say, either aloud or in your head, to inspire you in demanding situations. It can also help you process various scenarios and circumstances in life that may be outside your comfort zone, such as taking an exam, going to a job interview or participating in a sporting competition. Pep talks can be motivational or instructional – or even both: the goal is to encourage a positive outcome and boost your confidence.

The great thing about giving yourself a pep talk is that you don't need to rely on anyone else to deliver it: it's just there in your head whenever you need it. Being your own cheerleader is great for building up self-belief, too.

Try writing your own pep talk in the space below, choosing motivational phrases such as "You can do this" or "Your drive will see you through".

Make a confidence playlist

Most of us have songs that make us want to strut our stuff as soon as we hear them. Whether it's a taste of 1980s electropop or you like to get down with rap, songs that make you feel strong, confident and ready to take on the world should be in your daily playlist.

Perhaps the people who inspire you are musicians – can you channel their confidence or diva-like qualities and lyrics next time you hear the song? Use the space below to plan a confidence-boosting playlist.

Naming feelings

Naming the emotions that you're feeling is a powerful way of acknowledging you're human, and it's OK to feel a certain way. Studies have shown when you name what you're feeling, the feeling itself loses its impact and you become better able to control it.

For example, saying "I am angry" has a very different emphasis from "I feel angry." The former defines you as an angry person, whereas the latter helps you to recognize that you are not your feelings – you are more than that. While feelings come and go, our essence remains – which hopefully isn't "an angry person"!

Naming feelings in a non-judgemental way also helps to affirm your self-worth and opens the opportunity to regain power over them. Next time you need a bit of extra confidence, take a moment to name what you're really feeling – aloud, in your head or by writing it down.

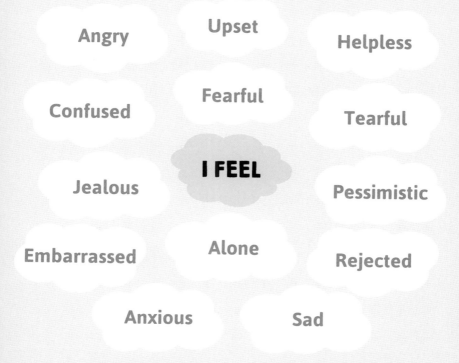

Angry Upset Helpless

Confused Fearful Tearful

Jealous **I FEEL** Pessimistic

Embarrassed Alone Rejected

Anxious Sad

What are you feeling right now?

How are you feeling right now?

Before you answer with the stock reply, "I'm OK," spend a moment digging a little deeper. How are you *really* feeling?

Identify your feeling or feelings and name them below. Remember to use "I feel…" rather than "I am…".

Confidence meditation

Make meditation your superstrength. Not only does medical research show that practising meditation can help reprogram the neural pathways in your brain, improving your ability to self-regulate your emotions, but it also calms you down by lowering your heart rate and blood pressure. All of this can have a positive impact on your self-confidence because if you're less stressed, you'll be in a more receptive frame of mind to allow positive thoughts to flow through you.

You can meditate anywhere that feels comfortable and where you won't be disturbed, but a quiet spot with a chair or cushions is a good place to try. Here's a meditation for confidence. Read it through first, then go through the steps one by one.

1   Get comfortable and set a timer for three minutes, or choose a relaxing song.

2   Close your eyes and pay attention to your breathing. See if you can slow it down a bit.

3   Imagine a beam of light shining from the top of your head.

4   The light fills you with confidence. Picture the light flowing downward until it's bathing your whole body.

5   Concentrate on your breathing and the feeling of light infusing you with confidence.

6   When the timer runs out or the song ends, slowly open your eyes.

Meditation works because it allows you to switch your thinking. If your mind is distracted by your breathing or visualizing an image, it doesn't have a chance to focus on negative thoughts and emotions. It's all about changing your state of mind and creating a positive space in your head that you can access if you begin to overthink a situation or if you're struggling with difficult feelings.

In the space below, note down how you're feeling now you've tried meditating. There are prompt words if you need them.

Calm   **Upset**

Relaxed

Anxious

Uncomfortable

Bored   **Energized**

Confident

Meditating isn't for everyone. If you haven't done it before, sitting alone with your thoughts can feel a little unsettling, but know that it's OK. Just like anything else, it takes a bit of practice to get the hang of meditation. If you feel it helped, then it might be worth sticking with it. If it's not for you, that's perfectly fine, too.

Listen to your thoughts

Sometimes it can be hard to tune out the world around you and enter the inner world of your thoughts. The buzz and noise of everyday life helps to keep you distracted and busy, and there's little time for introspection. This is sometimes a good thing in the short term as it helps to keep you focused on getting through the day, but it also means you spend hardly any time listening to yourself and what your mind is trying to tell you.

The reality is, if you're not paying attention to your thoughts, you aren't paying attention to your life. You're not really living your best life; you're just letting time pass. Your thoughts can help you to better understand your authentic self – your wants, needs, desires, even your anxieties – which is vital if you're going to build up your self-confidence. The aim is to wake up every morning *wanting* to live your best life and knowing you'll have a good day, rather than waking up and thinking "Urgh... not another day."

The way to shift this negative narrative is to start listening closely to your thoughts. What are they saying right now? When was the last time you analyzed their purpose and questioned them?

Take a moment to clear your mind of all other distractions and try writing your thoughts here, on scrap paper or in a notebook. You don't have to show this to anyone, so be as candid as you can.

The act of writing your thoughts down is cathartic: it helps you feel better about yourself because you can offload what you're thinking in a safe, non-judgemental space.

If your thoughts bring to light a lot of anxieties and worries, that's OK – you can put those to effective use. Writing down any self-doubt you have can help you to consider it from a more confident perspective.

Try this exercise: fill in the first column with any worries or self-doubt you're currently experiencing. In the second column, write what you'd say to yourself if your confidence were higher. You can try this exercise on a separate piece of paper if you feel you need some extra space.

Example: "I really need to pass my exam for my job, and I'm anxious that I won't. I'm not smart enough. I know I'm going to fail."

Example: "You've got this. You've done loads of revision, and your boss wouldn't have put you forward if you weren't ready. You've already passed three exams with ease and this one is no different. Just focus and breathe – you can do it."

Studies show that writing down your thoughts helps to reduce feelings of depression, anxiety and stress because it gives your mind a chance to organize and process them in a way that's difficult to do when they're stuck in your head.

If you've found that writing things down has helped, you'll find the section on page 94 (on how regular journalling can boost your self-confidence) of interest too.

What is mindfulness?

Mindfulness means connecting with the present moment. It's a simple but brilliantly effective concept that originated in Buddhist philosophy and has since become a popular holistic therapy due to its proven benefits, which include reducing anxiety, improving concentration and boosting confidence and self-esteem.

You can do anything mindfully – eating, walking in the park, stroking a pet; all you need to do is focus all your attention on the activity. For example, if you're strolling in the park, you might notice the way the wind is rippling through the grass, how the breeze is tickling your face, the pattern and texture of the bark on a tree, and how this makes you feel.

If a pet has just settled in for a cuddle, take it as an opportunity to be mindful by noticing the smell and texture of its fur, the warmth of its body and the emotions you feel. When your mind is focused in this way, it doesn't have time for anxieties or the negative thoughts that are prompted by low self-confidence.

How to be mindful

Practising mindfulness will help you to manage tricky moments in the future without being overly reactive or overwhelmed by what's going on around you.

Try these mindfulness exercises:

Mindful feet

Sit or stand with your feet touching the ground. It can be on any surface. Think about the soles of your feet. You don't need to look at them: just turn your attention to them. What can your soles feel? What sensations, temperatures and textures are you aware of?

Mindful walking

Head out on a walk and turn your attention to the world around you. What do you see, hear, smell and feel? Is the sun warming your face? What does the air feel like against your skin? When negative thoughts intrude, acknowledge them and then return to being mindful of your activity.

Mindful chores

Even scrubbing the dishes can be mindful – in fact, it's so boring, it is easy to get in the right mindset to be mindful! Use your senses to immerse yourself in the present moment. Inhale the scent of the washing-up liquid or feel the temperature of the warm water and the tickling sensation of the bubbles in the sink. When you catch your mind wandering, simply turn your attention back to what you are doing.

Pick a confidence role model

You probably know people who look like they've totally got themselves together and know what they're all about. Having a confidence role model can be quite useful for nurturing your own. Who would you choose? It might be a celebrity, a fictional character, someone from history, someone in the public eye or someone you know.

Write your confidence role model's name in the centre of the box below and brainstorm the words you associate with them – these might be adjectives, song lyrics, quotes or things they're well known for. This person has a new and important accolade – they are now your confidence role model. When you feel low in confidence, imagine they are with you, radiating courage and self-belief and guiding you to be your most confident self.

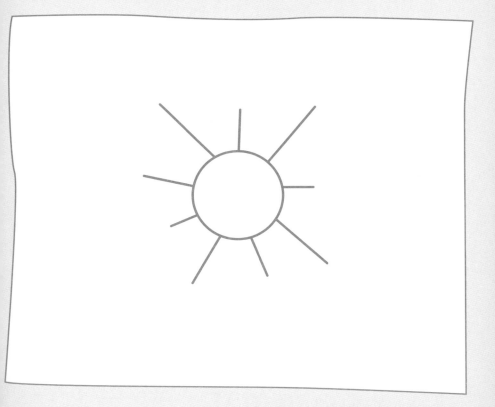

Twelve quick confidence hacks

1   Listen to your favourite music. Choose a song that makes you feel strong, confident and ready to take on anything.

2   Go outside. A change of scenery and fresh air on your face can snap you out of negative thinking patterns and make you feel calmer. You can also practise mindfulness as you walk.

3   Stretch then stand up straight. Stretching releases stress and tension in the body and mind, bringing you a rush of confidence. Check your posture, too. Now focus on standing up straight and walking tall for the rest of the day – you'll be amazed at the difference it makes to your confidence.

4   Give yourself a pep talk. Look in the mirror and remind yourself how capable you are. Use the motivational words on page 41 to help you get energized.

5   Have a cold shower. It may seem highly unappealing (especially in winter), but studies show that when you take a cold shower you initiate an antidepressant effect within your body that stems from activating your sympathetic nervous system. The chemicals that are released in your blood flood the mood-regulating areas of your brain with neurotransmitters and mood-boosting endorphins.

6   Doodle or do mindful colouring. A bit of random creativity calms the mind and helps you feel more in control. There are tons of adult colouring books on the market; just choose your favourite.

7   Take a deep breath. Oxygen boosts confidence by bringing energy and focus to your mind and body. Let your breath out slowly and, as you feel the air leaving your lungs, enjoy the sensation of calm.

8   Shake it off. Imagine you're shaking the self-doubt out of your body. Jump up and down, shake your arms and legs, roll your shoulders back. Anything that gets your blood flowing is a good physical and mental boost.

9   Hydrate. A glass of water clears your mind and makes your body feel instantly stronger and calmer. It also helps with focus and concentration levels.

10 Channel the confidence role model you picked on page 51. What would they do if they were faced with the same scenario?

11 Feel proud. Think of a time you achieved something amazing, to remind yourself how brilliant you are. It doesn't have to be mind-blowing – sometimes just getting out of bed can be worth celebrating.

12 Text a friend. Share your feelings with someone you trust and ask for words of encouragement.

Embrace being you

There are some days when you just don't feel yourself. Sometimes the reason is clear – perhaps you've had a disagreement with a friend or you're worrying about a forthcoming project – and you know the feeling will pass. But sometimes that state of mind lingers a little bit longer and you start to feel like everything is going wrong and that you're failing at life. You convince yourself that if you were more confident then everything would go right. If only you could change who you are.

It might feel like you need to transform into a different person to be confident, but that's not the case. True confidence is already part of you. It's about knowing who you are and understanding your identity: what you want and need in life (as well as what you don't need) and how to achieve it. It's also about calmly asserting yourself because you know your boundaries. It's saying "yes" and "no" with respect, but also with integrity and honesty. It's about surrounding yourself with people who make you feel good about yourself, but also knowing that not everyone is going to agree with you – and that's OK.

You can do all of this if you embrace your true, authentic self.

Self-confidence emergency kit

Here are some different ways you can get a quick confidence boost when you most need it. Sometimes, when you're not feeling at your most confident, it's hard to remember what helps, so it's good to prepare this toolkit in advance to steer you in the right direction whenever you need it.

You can use this page to write the things that give you a boost. You can come back to it whenever you need to.

I can talk to...

An idea that helps me...
(For example, "listen to what my thoughts are telling me")

An activity that helps me...
(For example, mindfulness)

Remember that...
(For example, "If I am being my true self, I am OK just as I am")

A song that makes me feel strong...

An affirmation that fills me with confidence...

PART 3
Overcoming self-doubt

Whether your confidence is high or low, it's natural to have moments when you doubt yourself. It's that niggly little voice in your head reminding you that you can't do something because you'll fail or that you don't deserve nice things because you're a rubbish person. You look around and it seems everyone else is breezing through life like they were born to succeed.

Think of your confidence role model from the previous section. When they walk into a room, people notice. They know the right thing to say at the right time. When they speak, people listen. On the face of it, they seem to have it all worked out – especially their confidence. You probably think they've never had an insecure thought in their lives. But even the most confident people have wobbly moments. The only difference is that they've learned to master their self-doubt and use it to reach higher, try harder and be stronger. Self-doubt is the enemy of self-confidence – its main goal is to make you feel awful, but you can drown it out by learning how to reset your mindset and being your very own cheerleader. You just need an open mind, a pen and a little patience.

Thoughts aren't facts

It's normal to think negative or critical thoughts occasionally. But when your self-confidence is low, you can get trapped in a loop of thinking those thoughts all the time. Not only is this damaging to your mental health, but often the things you're thinking aren't even true.

Self-doubt is learned. As you go through life, you are shaped by your upbringing, experiences and other people's opinions, meaning your confidence can be easily undermined by things that may be completely out of your control.

Often you believe things about yourself without questioning them, but just because you're thinking them, it doesn't mean they are a fact. Thoughts are just thoughts and facts are facts. The two are distinct and entirely separate from each other.

Next time that little negative voice pops into your head, try questioning whether it is true, fair or useful. If it isn't, simply acknowledge it and then move on.

Questions for your thoughts

The average person has approximately 6,000 thoughts every day. Some will be worthwhile ("I'm absolutely killing this project"), others not so much ("why am I such an idiot?"). But how many of these do you stop and question?

When you get caught in a cycle of negative thinking and self-doubting, it is useful to have a set of questions you can ask to establish whether you're being too hard on yourself. Try asking yourself:

- **Am I being fair to myself?**
- **Am I blaming myself for something I have no control over?**
- **Is it helpful to me to think this?**
- **Am I imagining the worst possible outcome?**

- **Is it likely to be true?**
- **Am I going to lose my job for making one mistake?**
- **Is it based on facts? For example, "I always fail" is not a fact.**
- **What facts prove this thought wrong? For example, "I have a good group of close friends".**
- **Would I say this to my best friend? If not, I shouldn't be saying it to myself!**
- **Am I going to allow this to dictate my mood for the rest of the day?**

You can think through these questions or write your answers out.

Speak as if you are confident

You can fake confidence to an extent. While the aim is for you to radiate natural confidence, there are certain things you can do to appear more assured. One of those is speaking with confidence – even if you don't feel completely confident inside.

The first thing to acknowledge is that it's not about *what* you say, but *how* you say it. A wobbly voice betrays nervousness, and when you are anxious your breathing often becomes shallower, which can affect the tone and cadence of your speaking voice. If you need to speak in a scenario you know you'll find uncomfortable, practise controlling your voice and try some relaxation techniques (such as mindfulness) beforehand. Turn to Part 4 to find more tips on how to act confidently.

Top talking-with-confidence tips:

- **Take deep breaths to slow your breathing down – this will help you slow your speech down too.**

- **When you're nervous you can speak too loudly or too softly – dial it down or up a notch if necessary.**

- **Keep a low pitch – a low, clear voice signals confidence, while a high voice signals nervousness.**

- **Don't be afraid to pause – it will give you a chance to take a breath, collect your thoughts and slow yourself down.**

- **If you're nervous, tell yourself this is a moment in time that will pass.**

- **Allow yourself time to relax before you need to speak.**

Becoming aware of how you speak requires patience and a little practice, but it's worth it. Almost all people who consider themselves to be confident individuals have also mastered the art of effective communication – not just in front of an audience but when speaking on a one-to-one basis, too.

While the delivery of what you're saying is important, having the strength of conviction to actually say it in the first place is also crucial. This comes from the self-belief you have within yourself, but you can also make yourself sound more confident by the language and phrases you use. Let's look at that more closely.

For example, if you say: "I think the process was challenging, but it was not without its rewards," it doesn't sound as impactful as if you'd simply said: "The process was challenging, but it was not without its rewards."

It may be a subtle change (taking out the words "I think") but it makes a dramatic difference. It doesn't sound forced or arrogant – it sounds natural, assertive and as though you have total belief in what you're saying, rather than trying to gain validation or approval from others.

Recap: If you start a sentence by saying "I think..." or "But maybe...", then any words you say following this lose their impact. If you just say the statement, it conveys the belief you have in your own words and sounds more convincing.

How past experiences affect your confidence

"Leave the past behind you" is a phrase most of us are familiar with. It encourages you to pick yourself up, get going and move on. It persuades you not to dwell on the negatives and certainly doesn't leave any room for wallowing in despair or engaging in self-reflection. But if you can find the courage to look back, you can learn from the past and break any negative patterns you've become trapped in – which is good news for your confidence.

Your past shapes who you are today and can have a profound impact – both positive and negative – on many areas of your life. When you experience a negative life event, your brain remembers your response and will try to protect you from going through the same emotional pain again. This means it's on high alert for any scenario that threatens you and is ready to react if it senses danger. That annoying voice of self-doubt is your brain trying to protect you from doing something that might hurt you. But it sometimes misfires, and if you believe what it's telling you then, you may miss an opportunity to do something amazing.

While you can't change what's happened in your past, you can use your past experiences to retrain your brain and write a new, confident story that draws on those experiences but doesn't allow them to negatively impact your everyday life. Over the next few pages, we'll be looking at how to keep your self-doubt in check.

How to respond to self-doubt

Self-doubt is normal. It's a protective mechanism that your brain uses to keep you safe. The problem is, it has a habit of doing risk assessments when they aren't necessary. It's like having a personal health and safety officer – except this one won't allow you to do anything out of the norm in case something bad happens. This is a problem because you need confidence to be able to challenge yourself in life, achieve great things and develop your skills and abilities, but self-doubt doesn't like any of that. It's quite happy just doing the same monotonous things inside its comfort zone, day in, day out, so when you want to push yourself to do something new or different, it tells you that you're not good enough or too stupid.

But there are things you can do to kick self-doubt back into its place when it's misbehaving:

- **Be kinder to yourself – we all make mistakes and that's OK.**
- **Remind yourself of your past achievements. We've all got something we're proud of, so use that as an example of how amazing you are.**
- **Don't compare yourself to others.**
- **Be mindful of your thinking and question your thoughts.**
- **Surround yourself with people who support you.**
- **Know your own beliefs and values and use them to cement the faith you have in yourself.**

Be your own cheerleader

Most of us have a cheerleader in our lives. They're the ones rooting for you loudly and proudly. They're there holding your hand when you're upset and they know exactly what to say to keep you on track.

The problem is, they can't be with you 24 hours a day. In the small hours, when anxiety hits and your self-confidence plummets, your cheerleader is likely to be in bed, fast asleep. Wouldn't it be great if you could have your own personal cheerleader living inside your head that could cheer you on whenever you need?

Great news: that person already lives in your head – it's you. You think nothing of cheering on your loved ones, yet thanks to your lack of self-confidence, you can be utterly useless at doing it for yourself. Time to change that with some cheerleading practice.

Start by focusing on positive things about yourself that you like and are proud of. Write down answers to the statements below to power up your inner cheerleader.

Five things I'm good at...

Five things I'm proud of...

Five things I like about myself...

If you're having trouble, use these ideas to get you started:

- **I'm a great friend**
- **I make people laugh**
- **I'm thoughtful**
- **I'm clever**
- **I'm a good listener**
- **I'm creative**
- **I'm honest**

Self-doubt circuit breakers

When you hear that nagging, critical voice creeping in, it's best to stop it in its tracks before it has a chance to do any damage. Next time you feel the negative thoughts getting louder, try one of these circuit-breaker exercises to help you concentrate on something else.

Pick an object to concentrate on, keeping your eyes still as you count to ten. It could be something on your desk, outside the window or in your house. When you concentrate on keeping your eyes still, your brain is too busy to access its full range of thoughts and emotions.

Stand up as tall as you can. Take a deep breath and puff out your chest. Relax your shoulders and spread your fingers wide. When you practise powerful, positive body language, you'll be sending messages to your brain to reinforce confident feelings.

Try alternate nostril breathing. Press down on your right nostril, breathing in for four seconds and out for four seconds through your left nostril. Then close the left nostril and follow the same pattern breathing through the right nostril. Repeat three times on each side. The deep breaths will boost your confidence, and keeping track of where your fingers need to be will distract your brain.

Stand with your feet flat on the floor and gently squeeze the muscles in your feet for five seconds and then release them. Then squeeze the large muscles in your calves for five seconds, then gently release. Next, squeeze your thigh muscles for five seconds before releasing. Keep going up your body with every muscle group. Concentrating on your body in this way helps take the focus off what's happening inside your head.

Never let self-doubt

hold you captive.

Roy Bennett

Write yourself confident

Every morning, try hopeful journalling to visualize the best possible outcome for your day. This technique really comes into its own when you've got a challenging day ahead of you because it allows you to think through workable solutions to the things you are worrying about, as well as prepping your brain to expect a positive outcome rather than a negative one.

Think about how you'd like the day to go, what feelings you'd like to experience, what you'd like to achieve and how you might do it. Be hopeful but realistic by setting your expectations at a level that feels comfortable rather than trying to aim too high – that way you can score some confidence-boosting easy wins. Look at it more like a wish list for the day and you can't go wrong. Try it by finishing the prompts below.

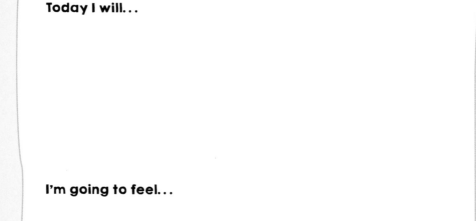

Today I will. . .

I'm going to feel. . .

I will achieve...

To do this, I will need to...

I will look after myself by...

Break-it-down planner

Sometimes life can seem a little overwhelming, especially if you're trying to achieve something different or important. Your voice of self-doubt tells you that it's too much and you're just not capable of seeing it through, and, before you know it, you've given up without even having started. Sometimes you just keep putting the task off because you're scared of failing. The problem is that the longer you put off beginning something, the bigger a problem it becomes, especially if it's something work- or college-related like a business report, essay or presentation, where there's a deadline.

But what if you break it down into smaller steps? Breaking down a large task into more manageable parts makes it easier to achieve. It gives you a confidence boost every time you complete another step towards your bigger goal, and, if you can see progress being made, you're much more likely to stick at it. Don't wait until you reach the top of the mountain before feeling proud of yourself: celebrate every step you take.

Think of a goal you're working towards. It can be anything – home improvements, a project at work or getting on top of life admin. Use this planner to break it down into steps. Make sure each step is specific (so you know when you've achieved it), realistic (so it doesn't feel overwhelming) and give yourself a time frame to achieve it in.

For example: "I want to sort out all my life admin and file it away alphabetically in the cupboard."

Break it down: spend a designated hour every day sorting through paperwork and shredding anything that isn't useful. Celebrate each day by giving yourself a cheer.

Part of achieving your overall goal is the knowledge that you can celebrate every step it took to get you there. Research shows that rewarding ourselves with a mini celebration helps us to stick to new habits because they create positive emotions. When we associate these new actions with positive emotions, we feel more motivated to do them. Next time you tick off a piece of life admin from your to-do list, why not give yourself a celebratory high five, do a victory dance or treat yourself to an episode of your favourite TV show?

Monday	Tuesday	Wednesday	Thursday	Friday

Next time you've got a big goal that's looking a bit scary, use the planner to break it down into manageable chunks so you don't give up at the first hurdle.

You can do this!

Big-goal planner

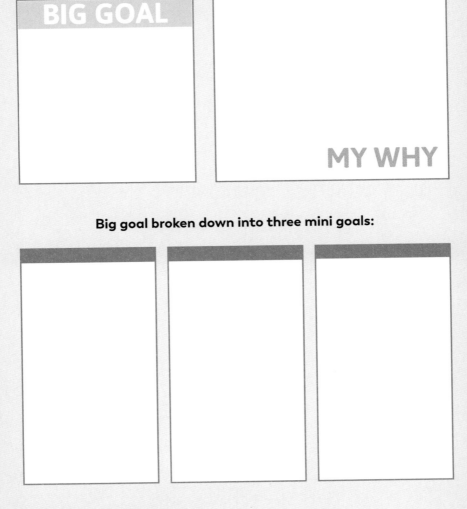

BIG GOAL

MY WHY

Big goal broken down into three mini goals:

Action plan to achieve mini goals:

	DATE:			DATE:			DATE:

PART 4

How to act with confidence

If you're not born with confidence, then where does it come from? Confidence is not something you have, like an arm or a leg, but it can be created – and that's where learning to act with confidence comes in. Being confident is nothing more than a feeling of certainty that you can accomplish or achieve whatever you set your mind to. So, it makes sense that if confidence comes from within, you can find ways to believe in yourself and boost your confidence at any time.

Creating a sense of self-belief doesn't mean all your problems will be solved, but it does mean that when you find yourself wandering off-track and things get tough, you can trust in yourself to manage the challenge and learn from the outcome. What's more, the longer you do this, the more natural it becomes, and you won't even notice that you were ever faking it in the first place!

Behaviours associated with low self-confidence

Low self-confidence is quite good at making itself known because it often shows up in our actions. You might relate to one or even all these descriptions. If that's the case, know that it's OK – and completely normal. We all behave differently in different situations and one person's comfort zone is someone else's idea of hell, so it makes sense that you might show avoidance in your behaviour one day but have high self-confidence the next.

Avoidance: avoiding or choosing not to do something because you're scared of failing or making a mistake. Because you don't believe in yourself, you often give up: at least then you can control the outcome.

Pete was the highest-performing sales consultant in his sector and was encouraged by his manager to apply for a more senior role. But his fear of interviews and giving presentations meant he didn't even want to try in case he messed it up.

Hiding: keeping your achievements and unique qualities a secret from others rather than embracing them.

Helen won a cross-country track event at the weekend. But she hid it from her friends and didn't put anything up on social media because she was worried they'd think she was a show-off.

Perfectionism: believing everything you do should be perfect and that nothing you do is ever quite good enough.

Jack was consistently late for work because he felt unable to leave the house unless everything was neat, tidy and put away in the right cupboards. He also fell out with his housemate, who had left a dirty bowl in the sink.

People-pleasing: trying to make sure everyone else is happy and calm, even if it means you're unhappy and stressed; the inability to say no even when the request compromises your own happiness and peace of mind.

A member of the events team at the college Akira attends asked her if she'd be able to help serve drinks at the next social event. Akira juggles college with a part-time job and caring for her elderly mother, but she wanted to show her support so said "yes". Now she is helping all the time and can't fit in any of the activities that help her relax, but she doesn't want to let anyone down.

Aggression: treating others in a bossy, threatening or bullying way; putting other people down to make yourself feel better.

When someone else makes a mistake at work, Joseph makes fun of them, but when Joseph makes a mistake, he gets angry and blames everyone else.

Attention-seeking: trying to get other people to tell you that you're a good or interesting person; trying to make people feel sorry for you; doing risky or shocking things so people take notice of you.

When Hannah joined her company, she told her new colleagues that she'd attended a prestigious university because she thought it made her sound clever. She's had to tell loads of lies to keep up the pretence, but she's worried that her colleagues would think she's stupid if they found out the truth.

Other signs of low self-confidence:

● **Struggling to accept compliments**

● **Worrying about what other people think of you**

● **Accepting the blame even if it isn't your fault**

● **Fearing being in charge or leading a team**

● **Backing down in arguments just to please others**

The truth is these behaviours often give you short-term relief in the moment and you feel a little better about yourself because you've dealt with whatever is making you afraid, but all you're really doing is allowing self-doubt to triumph. Remember, the more you let self-confidence win, the more positive experiences your mind will be able to draw from to keep self-doubt at bay.

Learning to act with confidence will take time, and you may feel uncomfortable, but by doing so you'll be giving yourself the best chance to change your life for the better.

Use the space below to describe a time when low self-confidence affected your behaviour.

If you could go back and relive that situation again, would you do anything differently?

Make changes by pressing pause

How many times do we wish we could have just taken a moment to pause, reflect, assess and then react? It's so easy in the heat of the moment to react hastily and fall back on your tried and tested means of dealing with a sticky situation. This probably looks all too familiar:

1   Something/someone triggers your emotions.

2   You react negatively.

3   Time passes.

4   You calm down.

5   You regret reacting negatively.

Recognize the scenario? You should do, because it's one that happens to all of us, at some point. But there is something you can do to lessen the impact in this type of situation and hopefully achieve a positive outcome: you can press pause.

Pressing pause means recognizing when you're in a situation that is making you feel like you want to react in a negative way. For example, perhaps your boss or college tutor criticized a piece of work you put a lot of effort into and it's made you feel angry. Or maybe you've let a loved one down and the guilt is making you snap at everyone around you.

If you're letting your emotions influence your behaviour, it's time to press pause.

Once you've recognized this, take a deep breath and acknowledge your thoughts and feelings – rather than rushing to make them go away. It may feel counter-intuitive, but you are safe to feel uncomfortable feelings, and they are often a sign that you're acting with courage.

How to press pause

1   Stop what you're doing (if it's safe to do so).

2   Put your hand on your heart and take a deep breath in and out.

3   Say to yourself (aloud, in your head or in writing): "I'm feeling..." e.g. scared, angry, guilty.

4   Notice where in your body you're feeling the emotion.

5   Notice your thoughts and remember that thoughts are not facts.

6   If you feel the urge to do one of the low self-confidence behaviours, you can say, think or write: "I really want to... but I won't."

7   Take three more deep breaths in and out. How do you feel after pressing pause? Those feelings of discomfort and the urge to act might not have gone away completely, but hopefully they will feel more manageable.

Be more assertive

Finding your voice can be hard. When you have low self-confidence, you convince yourself that what you have to say isn't worth listening to or that your wants and needs are somehow less important than everyone else's. Learning assertiveness can help fix this – because when you're being assertive, you're acting with confidence. Being assertive allows you to better manage your emotions as well as other people and situations. It is the ability to express your opinions positively and with confidence, while also respecting the views of others.

Hang on... isn't being assertive just being rude to get your own way?

Absolutely not, but it's worth recognizing there is a fine line between assertiveness and aggression, and people often mix them up. The main difference is that assertiveness is all about balance – you can express your own wants and needs, but you are also able to recognize and consider other people's feelings too. Aggression is about winning – it's a selfish use of power to get others to do what you want, without any regard for their rights, needs and feelings.

Tips to help you be more assertive

Learn how to say "no" – and if that doesn't feel comfortable, think of other phrases you could use instead, such as "that isn't going to work for me" or "thanks, but I don't think so".

Begin to practise daily rituals of putting yourself first. Need someone else to do the dishes so you can finally relax? Find that assertive voice and delegate.

If you've got a specific situation in which you need to be assertive, run through what you're going to say beforehand. For example, if you're planning to ask for a raise at work, try role playing with a partner or friend so you can get straight in your head what you want to say.

Don't forget what your body is saying too. Practise keeping a neutral expression in front of a mirror. Stand up tall and make eye contact.

Use "I" statements like "I feel..." and "I prefer..." rather than "you" statements.

Don't be afraid or ashamed to ask for help when you need it.

Believe in yourself and express it with conviction. Worrying about the opinions of others prevents you from being honest with yourself and other people. Being proud of who you are and what you stand for is a clear sign of self-respect.

Offer your own opinion while respecting that everyone's opinion counts.

It's OK to say "no"

You can get into a habit of saying "yes" to everything because often it feels easier to agree, even if you don't want to . When you have low self-confidence, you can find it difficult to recognize when your needs are as important as everyone else's. You may also struggle to express those needs and worry that you'll upset the other person if you say "no". This book is here to tell you that saying "no" is OK. There are no awards for being the person who always says "yes", because all that will happen is that people will take advantage of you and you'll burn out, which will be even worse for your self-confidence.

Learning how to say "no", so you can honour and respect your own needs, is a great skill to have in your self-confidence toolbox. In fact, saying "no" to an unreasonable request is the greatest act of self-respect.

Here's how to do it effectively:

- **Take your time with the decision so you can consider your own needs. Ask for more time if necessary.**

- **Get out of the mindset that "no" is a bad word!**

- **If it's a genuine request from a loved one, see if you can come up with a solution together or offer an alternative.**

Get talking

Having low self-confidence can sometimes make it difficult for you to communicate with other people. Perhaps you don't value your opinion enough to express it, or you're worried you'll trip over your words or say something stupid. Whatever the reason that's holding you back from saying what you want or need to say, if you can make yourself heard, you'll be giving your self-esteem an all-important boost.

The good news is you can act like you know how to communicate confidently – even if you're stumbling over your words inside your head. If you can deliver your message clearly, concisely and with conviction then you've got a good chance of being able to pull off a confident performance.

There is no conversation more boring than the one where everybody agrees.

Michel de Montaigne

Top tips for talking

Conversation is a two-way street, so try to find the balance between talking and listening. If the conversation slows down or you feel that you are talking more than you should, just ask the other person you're talking to, "What are your thoughts?"

If you're meeting someone for the first time or you don't know them that well, stick to neutral topics. This is where "small talk" (about the weather, what's on the menu for lunch or where they've travelled from) comes into its own. Small talk, while not the most interesting, is useful if you have low self-confidence as it allows you to stay in your comfort zone while you get to know someone better.

Use open questions that start with "why" or "how" as they invite a more detailed answer and allow the other person to participate fully in the conversation.

Make sure you are "active listening" – be alert and interested, and don't interrupt. Only then can you respond appropriately to what they're saying. If you find it difficult to think of something to say in response, try using neutral filler sentences, such as: "That's so interesting, I've never thought of it that way before."

Don't forget to smile and be kind.

Confidence action plan

We've looked at how what you say and how you say it leads to acting with confidence, and how this can help you build genuine confidence. Now it's time to put some thought into how this can work in a real-life scenario.

Think about a situation that causes you to feel low self-confidence – perhaps one you wrote about for an earlier activity? How could you use what you've learned to act with assertiveness and confidence? Write your ideas here – you could even write a script for yourself:

Example confidence script

If Rob asks me to take on a portion of his work, but I'm already working at capacity, I'll just politely say, "That doesn't work for me."

If he tries to make me feel guilty for not helping him, I'll say, "It's not my responsibility to help you and it's going to affect my ability to do my own work – which I'm not willing to compromise on."

If he still can't respect that, I'll speak to my manager.

Acting with confidence

If you need a quick reminder of how to act with confidence, here's what you need to know:

- Don't forget you can press pause if you're in a tricky situation.
- Find your voice so you can express your needs with confidence.
- Get comfortable with saying "no".
- Stand up tall.
- Be proud of who you are.

PART 5

Taking good care of yourself

Life doesn't always leave a lot of room for looking after yourself. In fact, if one of your roles requires you to care for other people, such as children or a vulnerable loved one, there's a good chance that self-care is a luxury that rarely gets squeezed in. Or perhaps you have a demanding and pressurized career that means finding time to take stock of what your mind and body need to stay healthy takes a back seat.

But imagine for a moment that self-care was one of your daily priorities – what would that be like?

A vital part of cultivating healthy self-confidence is looking after yourself, but low self-confidence can make this difficult if you feel you don't deserve to have time to look after your own needs, or you have trouble expressing them. Perhaps your sense of self-worth makes it difficult for you to want to look after yourself or you feel guilty for prioritizing your needs above your family's. But putting yourself first every now and again is far from selfish – it's crucial to your overall well-being, physically and mentally.

Read on to find out how to recharge those inner batteries and raise your confidence by taking time for self-care.

What's the difference between physical and mental health?

Physical health relates to the health of your body. While some aspects of your physical health are out of your control (such as genetic illnesses), there are lifestyle measures you can employ to help safeguard your future physical health. These include eating well, staying active, not smoking, getting enough sleep and only drinking alcohol in moderation. This is self-care for your body.

Mental health relates to the health of your mind. A state of mental well-being allows you to maximize your own potential and contribute to society. Its importance to your everyday life is recognized by the World Health Organization (WHO), which asserts that "mental health conditions can have a substantial effect on all areas of life, such as school or work performance, relationships with family and friends and ability to participate in the community."

Having a healthy mind allows you to make personal decisions and interact with others as well as learn new concepts and participate in new experiences. Mood, behaviour and thinking are all part of overall mental health, which is why things become so challenging if you're struggling to find balance in your life.

But physical and mental health do not operate completely separately. Physical illness or disability can affect your mental health, just as poor mental health can have an impact on your physical health, too. The nervous system links the brain to every part of the body, so when you do something that makes your body feel good – like exercising or drinking a glass of water – that good feeling includes your mind as well.

Stay hydrated

When you don't drink enough water, it's not just bad for your body, it's bad for your brain, too. The human body is made up of approximately 60 per cent water, so it makes sense that you need to stay well-hydrated if you're going to give your body and mind the best chance at staying healthy.

While it won't solve any real-life problems, having a glass of fresh water will give you an instant boost if you're flagging. If you're dehydrated, you can often feel sluggish and a bit headachy, and have trouble concentrating – which isn't the optimum state to be in if you're aiming to be confident. Staying hydrated also helps you to calm down if you're feeling anxious, which will make you feel that little bit more in control if you're having a difficult day. You should be aiming for 2 litres (3.5 pints) of water a day – that's approximately eight tall glasses.

If you struggle to remember to drink regularly during the day, use this as an excuse to treat yourself to a funky reusable bottle or a snazzy sports flask that you can keep with you during the day. Better still, get a personalized one printed with your favourite affirmation – a confidence and physical boost all in one!

Eat well

Being "hangry" (anger caused by hunger) really is a thing. If you don't eat well or don't eat enough, your blood glucose levels drop and your body releases hormones to keep you going. These hormones have a powerful effect on your mental state, making you angry, upset or anxious – which is exactly what you don't need when you're working on your self-confidence.

Eating well means making sure you have enough fuel in your body to keep you physically healthy. If you feel well in your body, you'll feel well in your mind, too. The best fuel for your body is a nutritious, well-balanced diet. According to the WHO, a healthy diet for adults contains protein, fruit, vegetables, legumes (e.g. lentils and beans), nuts and whole grains (e.g. unprocessed maize, millet, oats, wheat and brown rice) as well as a little sugar, fat and carbs.

Aim for three meals a day with healthy snacks in between. Snacks that are high in vitamins and release energy slowly will help you to avoid that hangry feeling.

Healthy snacks

- **Greek yoghurt**
- **Bananas**
- **Sliced peppers and houmous**
- **Berries**
- **Almonds**
- **Wholewheat crackers**
- **Toast with peanut butter**

Using a tracker is a fantastic way to plan your meals and make sure your body is getting all the delicious nutritional goodness it needs. Aim to tick all five fruit and vegetables by the end of the day – and don't forget that all-important water, too, to aid digestion and keep you hydrated.

Week of: _____	Breakfast	Lunch	Dinner	Snacks	Total Calories	Fruit and Veggies	Water
Monday							
Tuesday							
Wednesday							
Thursday							
Friday							
Saturday							
Sunday							

Calming journalling

Writing down your thoughts isn't just cathartic, it's a brilliant stress-management tool too. Studies have shown that putting pen to paper can help reduce anxiety, lessen feelings of distress and increase well-being – all of which is vital for nurturing healthy self-confidence.

There are many ways to journal and few limitations on who can benefit. You can begin journalling daily, weekly or whenever you need a self-care break from everyday life: simply choose the journalling method that works best for you.

Journalling gives you the opportunity to take a break and examine your thoughts and feelings. By putting them into writing, you're able to address your worries, release your emotions and clear your mind. A self-care journal is a safe space for you to get to know yourself better and unravel the feelings in your head without feeling misunderstood or judged.

Tips for calming journalling

- **For maximum benefit, make journalling a self-care habit. Try to commit to 10–20 minutes a day and tie it in with another habit that helps you to relax, such as listening to music or having a hot drink.**

- **Be candid with yourself – no one is going to read it unless you leave it somewhere obvious.**

- **Don't edit your writing – just let your thoughts flow.**

- **If old-fashioned pen and paper aren't your thing, there are now lots of apps and online options you can try.**

- **If your musings are looking a little negative, try to balance them with expressions of gratitude and positivity.**

- **Allow time for reflection. Perhaps look back to what you wrote the day before and see if you feel differently about it. Can you consider it more objectively?**

Use the next few pages to try journalling, using the tips from the previous page. Choose a prompt from the box if you're struggling to find the right words to start.

Describe your best day.

Describe a challenge you've recently overcome.

Write down three things you're grateful for and why.

Describe how life would be different if you had high self-confidence.

Write down what you want to achieve today and how you can make that happen.

Describe the last time you made yourself proud.

Unplug yourself

It's never been easier to feel connected. Whether it's online or via video or phone, staying in touch with the world and the people you love is part of life in the twenty-first century. Building a connection with others is great for your mental health, but there are times when it's tricky to find the balance between making the most of technology and allowing it to become intrusive.

Spending time away from your screen every day so that you can connect with yourself as well is a vital part of nurturing healthy self-confidence. It also gives your eyes and mind a break.

How do you like to unwind away from screens? Here are a few ideas, and some space to add your own.

- **Taking a walk**
- **Listening to music**
- **Listening to the radio or a podcast**
- **Reading or listening to a book**
- **Drawing**
- **Journalling**
- **Gardening**
- **Catching up with friends and family**
- **Enjoying a hobby**
- **Crafting**
-
-
-
-
-
-

Taking time away from your screen every day is brilliant for your confidence. It means you can spend time getting to know yourself, because if you know what you're all about, it's easier for you to feel self-assured. The digital world, particularly social media, has an annoying habit of distorting reality and making you feel like your own life compares unfavourably to everyone else's – which is bad news for your confidence. When you step away from screens, it's easier for you to appreciate what's good in your own (real) world.

Use the tracker to plan where you can fit screen-free time in each day. Write in your fixed weekly commitments first, and schedule off-screen time around it.

Sunday		Monday	
Tuesday		Wednesday	
Thursday		Friday	
Saturday		Notes/to do	

Exercise your mind

Giving your brain a workout is just as important as putting your body through its paces at the gym. Not only is it good for your overall well-being, it's also brilliant for building and maintaining cognitive skills.

Your brain never stops learning and growing as you age – a feature called brain plasticity – but for it to do so, you have to flex your brain "muscles" on a regular basis, just as you would with your body. Studies by the Harvard University-affiliated Institute for Aging Research found that embracing a new activity forces you to think and learn, and, if it requires ongoing practice, it can be one of the best ways to keep your brain healthy.

Learning something new, or challenging yourself with a spot of mental gymnastics, is also a fantastic way to build confidence as it gives you a sense of achievement – and the more you get comfortable with trying (and sometimes failing) at something new, the better your resilience will be. It'll help you in everyday life too because it enhances memory, focus and our ability to function daily.

There are many ways you can flex your brain "muscles". Have a look below for some ideas and see if you can turn them into a regular habit.

Train your brain with these activities:

- Try a jigsaw puzzle – the more pieces the better.
- Play cards – a study found that a quick game of solitaire or bridge can lead to greater brain volume.
- Learn a new language. According to experts, bilingualism can contribute to better memory, improved visual-spatial skills and higher levels of creativity.
- Learn a new skill... and then teach it to someone else. Learning something new helps to build new connections in your brain and teaching it to someone else helps you hone and develop those connections.

You could also try...

- Crossword puzzles
- Brain teasers
- Memory or strategy games
- Crafting/making something from scratch

Exercise your body

Movement gives you an instant boost because it helps to free your mind from negative thought patterns by bringing your attention to your body. When you're physically active, your brain produces endorphins – brain chemicals that reduce pain, increase happiness and calm your emotions. The good news is that only a small amount of exercise is needed to give you a rush of endorphins, so don't sign up to the next marathon just yet, unless you really want to! The most important thing is that you engage with an activity you enjoy, because then you'll be more motivated to keep doing it and hopefully it'll feel fun too, rather than a massive chore.

There are many different activities you can try, from dance classes to boxing, chair-based exercises to outdoor t'ai-chi, as well as the ever-popular swimming and running. The possibilities are endless.

It makes sense to build exercise and movement into your daily routine as part of an ongoing good self-care habit. Even if you only manage a ten-minute walk each day or weeding the garden, it will help regulate your emotions and boost your confidence. In fact, little but often can be more beneficial than two or three bigger exercise sessions spread over the week. See the next page for ideas to get your blood pumping, whether you're in the house or outside.

If you're at home...

- If you've got a soft surface and some tins of food or bottles of water to double up as weights, there's no reason you can't exercise in the comfort of your own home. There are plenty of yoga and exercise videos available online, for beginners all the way up to more advanced cardio workouts – see what suits you best and get moving.

- Cleaning, vacuuming, gardening, having a clear-out or building flat-pack furniture are all DIY jobs that involve movement, which means they all count.

- If you have mobility issues or find it difficult to stand or move about, you can search for a set of chair-based exercises online.

- Even simple things such as running up and down the stairs or doing seated bounces on a yoga ball in front of the TV will help to get your heart rate up.

If you're out and about...

- Walk more. Take a longer route home or park further away from the school or office.

- Grab some friends and play a game of frisbee, kick a ball about or even have a water fight in the local park – anything that gets you moving.

- Local sports centres often have a wide variety of activities on offer, many of which will be accessible to everyone.

- Running or walking in nature helps you connect to wildlife and can provide a welcome break from the hustle and bustle of everyday life.

Exercise tracker

Where could you fit physical activity into your daily schedule? Write your week's timetable down here and see where you can find time to exercise:

Monday	
Tuesday	
Wednesday	
Thursday	
Friday	
Saturday	
Sunday	

Once you've slotted exercise time into your schedule, you can use a chart like the one below to record each activity. After a week, look back and see how hard you've worked, which will give you a confidence boost and motivate you to keep going. Remind yourself to stay hydrated by ticking off every glass of water you drink, too. You can also include a goal for the week, such as walk 10,000 steps a day or doing two yoga sessions instead of one, to give you something to work towards.

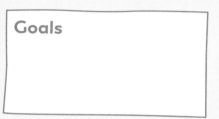

Goals

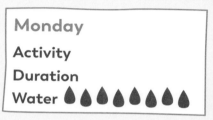

Monday

Activity

Duration

Water

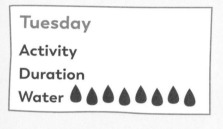

Tuesday

Activity

Duration

Water

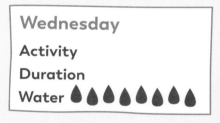

Wednesday

Activity

Duration

Water

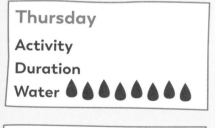

Thursday

Activity

Duration

Water

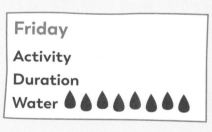

Friday

Activity

Duration

Water

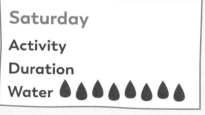

Saturday

Activity

Duration

Water

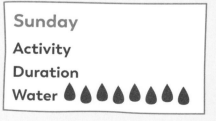

Sunday

Activity

Duration

Water

Yoga stretches

Yoga isn't just about physical strength and flexibility, it's great for your mind, too. Studies consistently show that yoga relieves stress, reduces anxiety and improves our overall mental health. Starting your morning with yoga will help you set a positive tone for the rest of the day and fill you with confidence. It can also help you relax after a busy day and get into a calm mindset for a good night's sleep.

Everyone can try yoga, irrespective of fitness or ability. Just take it at your own pace.

Have a go at these poses; then, if you enjoy them, why not try a class or go online for more inspiration? Try to hold each pose for 15 seconds (don't worry if you can't quite manage this).

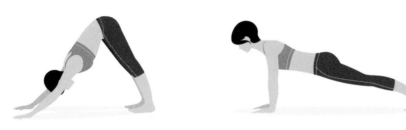

Downward-facing dog   **Full plank**

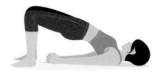

Bridge pose

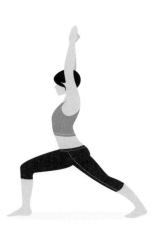

Warrior I pose

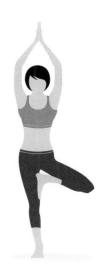

Tree pose

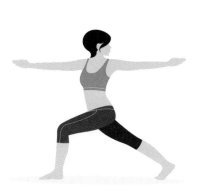

Warrior II pose

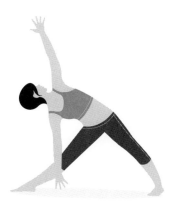

Triangle forward

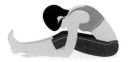

Caterpillar pose

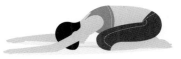

Wide child's pose

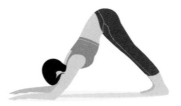

Dolphin pose

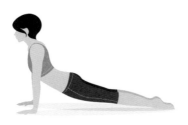

Upward-facing dog

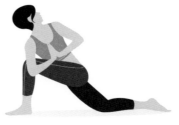

Revolved crescent lunge on the kne

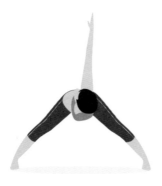

Wide legged forward bend V

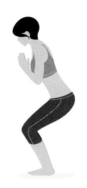

Chair with prayer hands

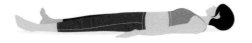

Corpse pose

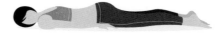

Front corpse pose

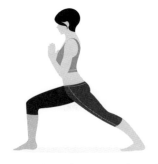

Warrior I with prayer hands

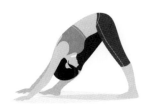

Pyramid with arms extended

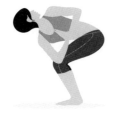

Revolved chair pose

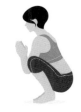

Garland pose

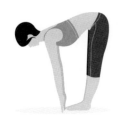

Halfway lift

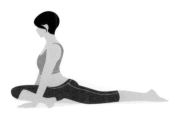

Half pigeon pose

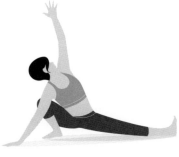

Side lunge with arms extended

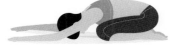

Extended child pose

Get into nature

Even if it's raining or gloomy outside, getting close to nature has been proven to increase feelings of positivity and well-being, two things you need in order to grow self-confidence.

Aim to get outside every day, if you can. Explore local green spaces, woods or a coastline, where you'll get the additional benefits of the peace and tranquillity that being close to water brings. If you can't go too far, you could try gardening. You don't even need a garden to grow flowers – just a windowsill, pots, compost and a bit of dedication. Growing food can also be extremely satisfying. It has the added benefit of providing a sense of achievement when you dish up a plate of home-grown, healthy fruit and vegetables at mealtimes.

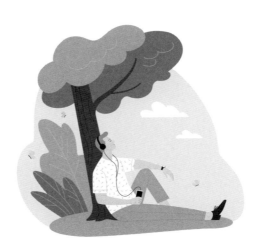

Top mood-boosting outdoor activities:

- Beachcombing if you're near the sea, or litter-picking for the ultimate feel-good factor
- Enjoying a picnic in your favourite place
- Stargazing
- Rambling or hiking in a group
- Wild cycling – exploring the countryside using bridleways, trails and tiny lanes
- Wild swimming – make sure you are in a safe place and don't go alone. See www.wildswimming.co.uk/health-safety for swim safety advice

If getting outside is difficult, don't forget you can bring nature into your home, too:

- Collect a selection of natural materials and create some artwork, or use them to decorate your living space.
- Create a nature nook by the window where you can watch wildlife – even if you're in an urban area, you'll be surprised by just how much you can see from a window.
- Find a comfortable spot and listen to nature sounds on a digital device – use it as a soundtrack to visualize an outdoor adventure.

A good night's sleep

Getting a decent night's sleep is the holy grail of well-being – who doesn't feel like they can take on the world if they're well-rested? But modern life likes to make it difficult for us. Stress, anxiety, ambient light coming in through the curtains, unruly children and pets, a restless partner, and feeling too hot or too cold are all things that love to interfere with your precious sleep. Lack of sleep can play havoc with your emotions and make you feel physically unwell, too. It can affect your concentration and memory as well as compromising your immune system, making you prone to illness and infections.

Bad-quality sleep is not going to boost your self-confidence – it's going to make it plummet instead. This is because it's harder for you to regulate your emotions when you're running on empty and the little daily challenges you may normally brush aside suddenly seem amplified – meaning that when your friend doesn't respond to the text you sent three hours ago, you start to get irritated for no good reason. This can then lead to feelings of self-doubt and a lack of confidence in yourself. The rule is: the more consistent your sleep cycle, the better you will feel. See the next page for some tips to help you establish a healthy sleep routine.

According to the National Sleep Foundation, adults aged 18–64 need 7–9 hours of sleep per night. Here's how to maximize your chances of getting all the sleep you need.

Prepare your sleep environment. Reduce noise and distractions and make sure your bedroom is warmer than 18°C but below 24°C.

Get your before-bed routine sorted. Turn screens off an hour before and pick up a book instead. Have a scented bath and get into some comfy pyjamas. It's less about the activity and more about giving your body signals that it's time to wind down.

Make sure you've had some fresh air and exercise during the day.

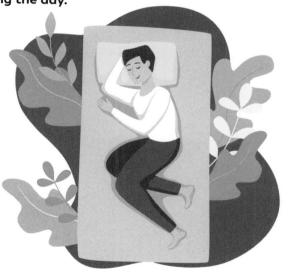

Try to go to sleep at the same time every night as it will help set your body clock. If you struggle to sleep, avoid napping in the afternoon or evening.

Recognize the importance of sleep. Don't party until the early hours or pull all-nighters for big projects. It might seem like a good idea at the time, but it will probably make you feel worse.

Avoid caffeine and sugary foods just before bed.

Sleep tracker

Try recording your sleep habits on the tracker below for the next week. Look for any emerging patterns so you can make any lifestyle adjustments to improve your sleep.

Today's date	Time I went to bed last night	Time I woke up this morning	How long I took to fall asleep last night	Total amount of sleep last night	How did I feel this morning? 1 – Wide awake 2 – Awake but a little tired 3 – Sleepy	What I did yesterday

Complete in the morning

Complete in the morning				
Today's date				
Time I went to bed last night				
Time I woke up this morning				
How long I took to fall asleep last night				
Total amount of sleep last night				
How did I feel this morning? 1 – Wide awake 2 – Awake but a little tired 3 – Sleepy				
What I did yesterday				

PART 6

Love your body

In an age of Photoshop, filters and social-media likes, it's hard to avoid comparing yourself to others. Your confidence can be linked to how you feel about your body, especially if you're being bombarded with images of "perfect" bodies – although it's important to remember perfect doesn't exist. If you're spending time worrying about how you look, you can forget how capable you really are, which can drain your confidence in the process. If you have low self-confidence, body image can be a particularly challenging topic. So when those doubts and insecurities creep in, how do you learn to love your own body?

It's easier than you think. Being comfortable in your body – however you think it looks – and not playing the comparison game are at the heart of healthy self-confidence. Your body is OK exactly as it is. Not convinced? Read on – the next few pages might just help change your mind.

The myth of "the perfect body"

Let's just put out there: there is no perfect body. Whether it's on the internet, social media, the TV or advertising, we are constantly being told what an (allegedly) perfect body is supposed to look like. If you have low self-worth and you don't trust your own values and opinions – which many people with low self-confidence don't – this can be a problem. It's easy to fall into a trap of believing everything you see and read, and before you know it, that little voice of self-doubt is winning the battle again.

But know this: your body is fine as it is. What's important is that you stop looking for imperfections and start celebrating how amazing your body truly is.

Beauty begins the
moment you decide
to be yourself.

Coco Chanel

Affirmations for body confidence

Having confidence in your body means you're happy in your own skin, whatever your size or shape. If you're not at peace with your body, you'll probably find you won't be at peace in your mind either. Of course, some days you'll feel more confident than others, but what you really need and deserve is to feel body confident all the time – and using affirmations can help with that.

Try reciting these affirmations to yourself. You could even write them on a sticky note and put them on a mirror. There's space for you to write your own, too.

My body is a gift.

I will accept my body, just the way it is.

I make healthy choices for my body because I respect it.

I choose self-love over self-criticism.

I am worth more than my appearance.

I am enough.

I am grateful for everything my body allows me to do.

If my body speaks, I listen.

I will not compare my body to other people's.

Keep a gratitude journal

To really feel the benefits of gratitude, you have to truly live it and believe it. Performing daily acts of gratitude can have a significant impact on your mindset and self-confidence, and can also help to cement positivity in your life. One of the best ways you can do this is to practise gratitude journalling. Even if you just spend ten minutes a day writing in your journal, it can give you a mood boost that takes your day from "OK" to "great" on a regular basis.

Try writing in this gratitude journal every day for a week:

Monday

I'm grateful to my body for...

_____

A person I'm grateful for...

_____

I'm grateful that...

_____

Tuesday

I'm grateful to my body for...

_____

A person I'm grateful for...

_____

I'm grateful that...

_____

Wednesday

I'm grateful to my body for...

A person I'm grateful for...

I'm grateful that...

Thursday

I'm grateful to my body for...

A person I'm grateful for...

I'm grateful that...

Friday

I'm grateful to my body for...

A person I'm grateful for...

I'm grateful that...

Saturday

I'm grateful to my body for...

_____

A person I'm grateful for...

_____

I'm grateful that...

_____

Sunday

I'm grateful to my body for...

_____

A person I'm grateful for...

_____

I'm grateful that...

_____

If your body is long overdue a "thank you" for all the hard work it does, try this body gratitude worksheet to show your appreciation.

Body gratitude worksheet

I am grateful for this body.

It helps me _____

This body is _____ **and** _____

It allows me to _____

_____

My face radiates _____

My eyes are filled with _____

My lips help me _____

My chin is _____

My neck holds me with _____

I am grateful for hands that _____

I am grateful for arms that _____

With this stomach I can _____

These hips help me _____

These legs allow me to _____

My feet are _____

Dress for confidence

Clothes are one of the best forms of self-expression. You may have to wear a uniform or follow a dress code at work or school, but in your own time, anything goes. Perhaps your go-to outfit is high heels and a cocktail dress, or you're at your best in jeans and a T-shirt. When you love the outfit you're wearing, it really shows because you'll be walking tall and strutting your stuff.

If you're concerned about body image, you may say that you'll wear a certain outfit when you lose weight or fit into a smaller size. But why wait? If you know wearing a particular outfit will make you feel awesome, start wearing it now.

Go into your closet and throw out all the items of clothing that make you feel bad about yourself. There is no place in your wardrobe for that oversized frumpy T-shirt you're keeping for emergencies but makes you feel utterly despondent whenever you put it on. Instead, wear clothes that make you smile and help you to love your body.

Just remember that, ultimately, dressing is always about attitude, feeling comfortable and confidence.

Kate Moss

Self-care toolkit

The self-care that works for you will be different from the next person's. Learning to love yourself is a personal thing and the activities you choose to help you feel good might differ day to day depending on how you're feeling.

Write about the things you can do daily or weekly. Don't forget to include the self-care you can show yourself when you need an extra boost. There are some suggestions below, but only add what works for you.

Every day I can...
For example: "Take a hot bath, do 10 minutes of gratitude journalling, say an affirmation"

_____

_____

Every week I can...
For example: "Get into nature, make time for a hobby"

_____

_____

When I need a boost of confidence, I can...
For example: "Give myself a pep talk, do some exercise"

_____

_____

When I want to show myself extra care, I will...
For example: "Grab a blanket and watch a movie, take a break from social media"

_____

_____

You can fall in love with your body – it'll just take a little time and commitment. Try some of these to see if you can build a good relationship with your physical self.

- Write down at least five things you love about your body; then, whenever you're having a low-self-confidence day, take out the list and remind yourself how fabulous you and your body are.

- Remove body-shaming triggers from your life – whether it's something on social media or TV, remember it's a distorted reality.

- Find an exercise class you enjoy and embrace moving your body.

- Be your own best friend – you wouldn't tell a friend they look horrendous today, so why are you doing it to yourself?

- Find your tribe. Good friends are like gold dust so surround yourself with loving people who don't make you feel bad about yourself.

PART 7

Be true to yourself

Sometimes it's easier not to stand out. When you stay incognito, you blend in with those around you. If you lack confidence in your value and self-worth, the temptation is often to just slot in with what you think everyone expects you to be. But by doing so, you sacrifice a little of yourself every time and lose a sense of what makes you, you.

Having healthy self-confidence is about knowing you can rely on yourself – every single time. It's about knowing what's important to you, what your boundaries are and what values you stand for. Quite simply, it's about being authentic and true to yourself. Read on for advice and tips for how to achieve just that.

What are boundaries?

Boundaries are rules, set by you, about how other people can treat you. They're different for everyone and they're a way of communicating with confidence what's OK and not OK for you personally. They can protect your physical as well as mental space and define the emotional limits of the relationships that you have with those around you. Research shows that when you have healthy boundaries, you develop your individuality and your own unique interests and skills – which is crucial for nurturing your sense of self and overall well-being.

Some examples of expressing boundaries could be:

- **"That doesn't feel comfortable for me, please stop."**
- **"I don't allow people to speak to me in that way."**
- **"That's not something I want to share with you."**
- **"You're standing too close – please move back a step."**

Only you get to decide what you will and won't do with your body, what kind of conversations you're comfortable having and how long you stay in any situation. Setting boundaries is empowering and lets other people know your limits respectfully, without compromising the relationship. If the other person genuinely cares about you, they'll respect you for it, as well as expecting you to respect their boundaries in return. As American therapist Elizabeth Earnshaw puts it: "When people set boundaries with you, it's their attempt to continue the relationship with you. It's not an attempt to hurt you."

When we have boundaries in place...

Healthy boundaries allow each person in a relationship or group of friends or family to communicate their wants and needs while simultaneously respecting the wants and needs of others. Examples include:

- **Being able to say "no" with confidence and accepting when someone else says "no".**
- **Respecting other people's values, beliefs and opinions, even if they are different from your own.**
- **Being able to clearly communicate your wants and needs.**
- **Honouring and respecting your own needs as well as the needs of others.**

When we have an absence of boundaries...

A lack of boundaries can lead to conflict and too much compromise. You might need to put boundaries in place when:

- **You're struggling to say "no".**
- **You're having trouble accepting "no" from others.**
- **You feel unable to communicate your needs and wants.**
- **You compromise personal values, beliefs, and opinions to satisfy others.**
- **You feel you're being manipulated into doing something you don't want to do.**

Remember: unhealthy boundaries often lead to unhealthy relationships that can become abusive in nature. Abuse – whether physical, sexual or emotional – is a violation of boundaries. If you need help, see the resources section at the back of this book.

Tips for setting boundaries

We've already looked at assertiveness on page 81 – now it's time to put it into action. Boundaries give a clear signal to the people in your life with regard to what you find acceptable and what you don't. They're a bit like stop signs that help you establish when a line has been crossed.

Setting boundaries is fundamental to your self-confidence. It often provides the balance you need to have successful relationships with friends, family and loved ones – as well as balance in your own life. Here are some examples:

Setting boundaries can help you to avoid doing too much for others. Sometimes it's difficult to say "no", particularly to a loved one, but when you end up doing too much for other people, resentment quickly sets in. Help them find support in other ways if you can.

Sometimes you need to set boundaries with yourself, too – such as knowing when to listen to your body and rest or knowing when you're at risk of overeating or having too much alcohol. Respect yourself enough to know your own limits.

How to set boundaries

- **Be clear exactly what your wants and needs are and convey them as concisely as you can.**

- **Start small and build up your confidence. Focus on one boundary at a time, particularly if you're attempting to shift relationship boundaries. If someone gets angry and tries to make you change your mind about a boundary, that's a sign you were right to set it and you should not back down.**

- **Have a goal. Ask yourself what you want to achieve by setting a boundary.**

- **It's OK to rethink a boundary if you want to give someone a second chance. Sometimes you can trust your gut, and if it feels right to give them another try, then do – remember, you're in charge.**

- **Write out what you want to say (you can use the space below) and practise in front of a mirror before you do it for real.**

- **Keep it simple and straightforward. Rather than overloading someone with too many details, pick the main thing that is bothering you and focus on that.**

Use the space below to jot down the boundaries you would like in your life, using the tips above. Think about your goals. You could even try scripting some boundary-setting statements so you can deliver what you want to say with total confidence.

What are your values?

There is much to value in having values. Values give your life meaning because they help to define who you are. Everyone has different values because the beliefs and qualities that are important to you may not be as important to someone else. The consensus among psychologists is that if you embrace values in your life, it helps you to feel genuinely happy and fulfilled because you're being true to yourself.

Sometimes you have a clear idea of what your values are – perhaps you prize honesty or a strong work ethic – but sometimes you might need a little help to work out what's important to you. Ironically, when it comes to values, the doubts you have about your own abilities are your friends. You need to listen to that annoying little self-doubt voice for a minute to hear what it's telling you. If it's nagging you about something, you can use it as a signpost to the areas in your life where you need to focus your values. If you feel that life is a bit dreary, then try building passion and excitement into your plans. Or if you're struggling to achieve your goals and your mind is telling you you're inadequate, then nurturing determination and resilience will help.

What are the core values that guide your life?

Circle the core values that resonate with you and add your own if you want.

Achievement

Adventure

Ambition

Courage

Charity

Dependability

Creativity

Education

Determination

Empathy

Faith

Family

Friendship

Fun

Generosity

Health

Hard work

Independence

Honesty

Integrity

Intelligence

Justice

Learning

Kindness

Loyalty

Love

Peace

Open-mindedness

Respect

Popularity

Security

Simplicity

Spontaneity

Success

Teamwork

Truth

Understanding

Wealth

Can you narrow your core values down to just three? Once you've chosen three that are most important to you, try putting each one in a statement that sums up why you value that quality.

Example: Determination

I value determination in myself and others. I refuse to give up when things get tough and will do my best to change a challenging situation into an opportunity for triumph.

_____

_____

_____

_____

_____

_____

_____

Having a reference point like this is a valuable tool for building self-confidence. It helps you to cement how you feel about the world and the people around you – which is vital for living your life as authentically as you can. Your values can change a little over time, but know that if life throws a curveball your way, you can always turn to your values to show you what to do.

Don't compare yourself to others

Most of us don't exist in isolation, which means we're very aware of how other people live their lives. Social media has made it all too easy for us to have a snoop into what other people get up to, such as what they do in their job, their hobbies, what they've achieved, their family life, where they go on holiday or what they do with their friends. This level of information-sharing makes it impossible for you not to compare your life to other people's – and if you feel you're falling short, it can be disastrous for your self-confidence.

But who sets the benchmark? Did someone wake up one day and decide that unless you style your hair a certain way or you're the CEO of a FTSE 100 company, you're failing at life? Measuring your appearance, strengths or achievements against other people's will inevitably leave you feeling bad about yourself, because there's always someone doing better than you – even if you are a CEO or have great hair, or both.

Expectations are often constructed by yourself and this means you can change them. You can do that by becoming more accepting of who you are and show yourself compassion. When you're kinder to yourself and recognize your own skills and abilities, you don't need to compare yourself to others.

Remind yourself of how amazing you are now. Without overthinking it, write down three things that make you, you.

What makes a good relationship?

Your self-confidence and how you feel about yourself are inherently linked to your relationships with the people around you. Consider your romantic relationships, for example. If you've had the misfortune to become involved with someone who's a little toxic and puts you down, the knock-on effect on your confidence levels can be profound, which can then affect other areas of your life, too. Similarly, your early life and upbringing, particularly the relationship you have with close family members, can influence your sense of self-worth.

When you think about the people who are important to you, there are certain things you can look for in a person to help you work out if they're destined to have a positive or negative impact on your life. This can help you decide whether you want them around (because they love and support you) or whether you might feel better about yourself without them.

You may not be able to choose your family, but if they're having a harmful impact on your self-confidence, there are steps you can take to limit their influence (see the next page).

Positive characteristics	Negative characteristics
Lets you be yourself	Puts you down for who you are
Lets you choose your friends	Controls who you see
Replies to your messages	Ignores or ghosts you
Is considerate of your feelings	Treats you like your feelings don't matter
Is interested in your thoughts, feelings and experiences	Only talks about themselves
Makes you feel safe	Makes you feel anxious and unsafe

Laughs with you	Laughs at you
You can tell them if they've upset you	Refuses to acknowledge they've upset you
They want to hang out with you	They will drop you for other plans

Damage limitation

Low self-confidence can make it hard to spot signs that a relationship has gone sour, particularly if the other person has made you think your feelings don't count. If you're in a friendship or relationship where you feel unsafe, uncomfortable or like you can't end it, it's not your fault and you're certainly not alone.

Talk to a trusted friend or family member about the situation. Then check out page 150 for more resources. You're not alone and you deserve to be treated with respect.

Remember...

You can take the risk of losing the relationship. If you've expressed how someone is making you feel and they don't value the relationship enough to change, you will have lost nothing by walking away.

Create boundaries and commit to them. For example: "When you say things like that, it makes me feel uncomfortable. Please stop or I'll leave." Be prepared to have your boundary tested and always follow through.

Know that having a friend or partner is not always better than having no friends or no partner. The best friend you have is you. Or, in the words of Taylor Swift, "sometimes in life you have to be your own best friend."

Confidence for life

Having good people in your life will help safeguard your self-confidence for a lifetime. Finding your tribe is like winning the relationship lottery – they'll be your cheerleaders, support and respect you. They'll pick you up when you're down and forgive you when you do something silly. Most importantly they'll love and care for you no matter what. The more you surround yourself with the right people for you – those that show all these qualities and more – the more confident you'll become in recognizing what you value in future relationships.

Sometimes you will lose friends along the way; it's all part of life, and it's possible a handful of people in your life might react badly as you grow in confidence and assertiveness. This is often a blessing in disguise because it's a quick way to tell who respects you and who doesn't. And if they don't? Well... you know what to do.

Find a group of people
who challenge and inspire
you, spend a lot of time
with them, and it will
change your life.

Amy Poehler

PART 8

Looking forwards

No one can predict the future, but that's what makes life exciting! Taking a big, or even small, step into the unknown can be scary, but it also presents you with the perfect opportunity to shape your own future. If not knowing what's around the corner is something you find difficult, planning and setting yourself a goal might be just what you need to help you maintain a positive mindset and stay in the high-self-confidence zone. Curveballs will always come your way, but if you can learn to deploy some defensive moves using self-confidence as your guide, you'll be much better at dodging them.

Maintaining healthy self-confidence is a lifelong project. You will never reach the point where you stop growing and developing, and your self-confidence will change to reflect that. But with the right support and a little self-help, you'll have fewer days feeling bad about yourself and more days knowing that you are amazing and are living your best life.

Goals for the future

Most mental health experts agree on one thing, and that is that setting goals for the future is a fantastic way to maintain a positive mindset and effect change in your life. Having a goal helps to keep you motivated and your mind focused on achieving your objectives, which is good news for your self-confidence.

All goals need a strategy, whether they are big (starting your own business) or small (clearing out the "drawer of doom" in the kitchen). Your goal might be related to yourself, such as growing your self-confidence, or it could be a skill or task you want to accomplish. Use the tracker on the next page to write your future goals and how you might break them down into manageable steps.

Be SMART

The best way to set a goal is to make them as SMART as possible:

Specific (For example: *"I want to be more confident in social situations"*)

Measurable (For example: *"I'll know I'm growing in confidence if I can chat to two people I don't know at the next work social event"*)

Achievable (For example: *"I can practise confidence skills to help me in the week before the event"*)

Realistic (For example: *"I don't want to feel nervous around my peers at the next social event"*)

Time-limited (For example: *"By the end of this year, I want to be able to enjoy all work events without feeling nervous"*)

Goals for the future

Goal	Start date		Actions
_____ _____ _____ _____	Finish date	☐ ☐ ☐ ☐ ☐	

Goal	Start date		Actions
_____ _____ _____ _____	Finish date	☐ ☐ ☐ ☐ ☐	

Goal	Start date		Actions
_____ _____ _____ _____	Finish date	☐ ☐ ☐ ☐ ☐	

Goal	Start date		Actions
_____ _____ _____ _____	Finish date	☐ ☐ ☐ ☐ ☐	

You're not alone

If you're having a tough time with self-confidence, you're not alone. People from all walks of life struggle with low self-confidence. Here are some of their stories:

I work in a pressurized environment and the culture is very much "stay late or find another job." I accepted this when I was younger, which was wrong with hindsight, but I felt fortunate to have gained a position in a prestigious company and I didn't want to lose my job. I'd always had low self-confidence and didn't feel I could speak up. But once I had a family, and I was losing precious time with my son because of working late (for which I wasn't even getting paid), I felt enough was enough. I had to find my voice for the sake of my child. He gave me the motivation I needed to find the confidence to start saying "no" and putting my needs first. I knew I'd done the right thing when one of the other parents at work said that I'd given them the confidence to do the same.

Jenny, 42

I've always been the quiet one in the corner - I'm not ashamed to say it, I'm a bit nerdy! I used to think there was something wrong with me - that I was boring, and I should be more outspoken, confident and self-assured like other men my age. I've always struggled to find like-minded people that I can really gel with, but I've recently found my tribe and I couldn't be happier. We mostly chat online, as that suits us all (some of us find social situations stressful), but they've helped me realize and accept that being an introvert is a wonderful part of who I am, and I should celebrate it.

Alex, 19

I'd always loved watching ballet as a child, so when I noticed the local dance studio was running adult ballet lessons I jumped at the chance, even though I'd never tried it before. When I got there, I could tell that everyone had done ballet when they were younger. They already knew all the positions of the feet, while I could barely keep my balance. At one point I fell over - I was mortified and vowed never to go back. All my confidence just disappeared, but this was something I really wanted to do and I hate giving up on anything. The dance tutor called me the next day to check I was OK and offered to give me a few one-to-one lessons just to get me up to speed. We're working on my confidence and my tutor says I'm ready to do group sessions as I've improved so much.

Kalani, 25

Ask for help

If you're struggling with low self-confidence or any other aspect of mental health, there are many organizations out there that can provide help and advice. If you feel like your confidence issues are becoming unmanageable and are starting to have a negative impact on your day-to-day life, you should speak to your doctor or healthcare provider.

British Association for Counselling and Psychotherapy (BACP)

www.bacp.co.uk

BACP's self-esteem pages explain how CBT therapy can help with confidence and self-esteem. They also include information about finding a therapist and personal stories.

Mental Health America

www.mhanational.org

Text "MHA" to 741741 to connect with a trained crisis counsellor. The website offers practical advice and support for all aspects of mental health, including links to online communities and tools for long-term wellness.

Mind (UK)

0300 123 3393

www.mind.org.uk

Find comprehensive information and support pages, as well as tips for living with anxiety, low confidence and self-esteem, depression and other mental health conditions. The website also includes an online community and a crisis resources page with self-help advice to help you cope.

The National Association for People Abused in Childhood (NAPAC) (UK)

0808 801 0331 / support@napac.org.uk

www.napac.org.uk

A traumatic upbringing or start to life can have a profound impact on our self-confidence. NAPAC supports adult survivors of any form of childhood abuse through a helpline, email support and local services.

National Domestic Violence Hotline (USA)

1.800.799.SAFE (7233) or text "START" to 88788

www.thehotline.org

Call for free confidential and compassionate support, crisis intervention information, education and referral services.

Refuge (UK)

0808 2000 247

www.refuge.org.uk

This is the organization to turn to for advice about domestic abuse and support for those affected by it.

Samaritans (UK)

116 123

www.samaritans.org

Samaritans provide mental health support and a listening service for those who wish to speak to someone confidentially and without judgement. Their lines are open 24 hours a day, seven days a week.

Samaritans (USA)

1 (800) 273-TALK

www.samaritansusa.org

Samaritans provide confidential and judgement-free hotlines for those who are struggling with their mental health or contemplating suicide. Their lines are open 24 hours a day, seven days a week.

SANE (Australia)

1800 187 263

www.sane.org

Information and crisis support are available for people with mental health challenges and their families.

Conclusion

Working on yourself is never easy because it involves being honest about how you're really feeling and admitting there are things you're not happy with and want to change. Congratulations on the progress you've made so far – hopefully, you're beginning to see a difference in your self-confidence and your mindset.

Nurturing your self-confidence is a commitment you need to make to yourself in the long term, but if you are prepared to be patient and use the resilience that's already inside you, you'll be giving yourself the best possible chance of succeeding. It needn't be too time-consuming either. The key is to make simple but effective changes, like the ones we've looked at in this book, and you'll be on your way to a confident future in no time. Go at your own pace, and, if you're not feeling it, try again another day – this book will be here waiting for you. You can make mistakes and know you're strong enough to overcome them. If you need extra help, reach out to the people you trust and let them help you, or seek professional help – you never need to suffer alone. You're confident, you're capable and you've got this!

Confidence is key –
once you have that,
you are unstoppable.

Timothy Weah

Resources

As well as the organizations detailed on pages 150–152, here are some further sources of inspiration and support that you can refer to during your confidence journey.

Websites

Positive Psychology (Netherlands)
www.positivepsychology.com/category/the-self/
Insightful articles, research and printable worksheets/activities designed by therapists for working on your self-confidence at home.

Psychology Today (USA)
www.psychologytoday.com/gb/basics/confidence
A comprehensive catalogue of self-confidence articles and tips, written by qualified therapists and counsellors.

Healthdirect (Australia)
www.healthdirect.gov.au/self-esteem
Tips and advice for working towards confidence and self-esteem.

Podcasts

The Confidence Coach with Cass Dunn
Clinical and coaching psychologist Cass Dunn speaks to real people struggling with their self-confidence and offers advice and techniques to tackle the problem head-on.

The Confidence Podcast with Trish Blackwell
The Confidence Podcast is the podcast for women who struggle with perfectionism, self-doubt and a self-critical voice.

The Self-Esteem and Confidence Mindset with Jonny Pardoe
A podcast for busy professionals wanting to boost their confidence to grow in their career/business and not hold back any longer.

Books

The Confidence Kit: Your Bullsh*t-Free Guide to Owning Your Fear (2018)
Caroline Foran

The 50 Secrets of Self-Confidence: The Confidence to do Whatever you Want to do (2015)
Richard Nugent

Eliminate Negative Thinking: How to Overcome Negativity, Control Your Thoughts, and Stop Overthinking (2020)
Derick Howell

Know Your Worth: How to Build Your Self-Esteem, Grow in Confidence and Worry Less About What People Think (2021)
Anna Mather

Online forums, support groups and communities

www.sidebyside.mind.org.uk (UK)
Mind's online community, where you can talk about your mental health and connect with others who understand what you are going through.

www.mentalhealthforum.net/forum (UK)
A friendly peer support forum for people experiencing mental health issues.

www.healthunlocked.com/anxiety-depression-support (USA)
Run by the Anxiety & Depression Association of America (ADAA), this online community is a safe space for those affected by anxiety and depression.

www.anxietycanada.com/resources/mindshift-cbt (Canada)
Download the app for access to the forum, where you can share stories and learn from others' experiences in a supportive and safe environment.

www.saneforums.org (Australia)
A supportive online community where you can chat with others in similar situations.

www.beyondblue.org.au/get-support/online-forums (Australia)
Online support for those living in Australia to achieve their best possible mental health.

Other titles in the series

The Anxiety Workbook

Practical Tips and Guided
Exercises to Help You
Overcome Anxiety

Anna Barnes

ISBN: 978-1-80007-397-5

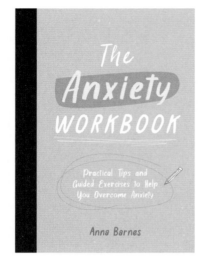

The Anxiety Workbook contains practical advice, effective tips and guided exercises to enable you to recognize and process your anxiety. Based on trusted techniques and mindfulness exercises, this guide will allow you to better understand your anxiety and will provide the tools you need to work through it.

The Self-Esteem Workbook

Practical Tips and Guided
Exercises to Help You Boost
Your Self-Esteem

Anna Barnes

ISBN: 978-1-80007-716-4

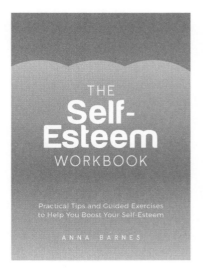

A healthy self-esteem is key to having a good sense of well-being, but it can often be challenging to feel good about who we are. This workbook contains practical advice, effective tips and guided exercises to help you build your self-esteem. Based on trusted CBT techniques, it will help you to grow your confidence and achieve long-term self-belief.

Have you enjoyed this book?
If so, why not write a review on your favourite website?

If you're interested in finding out more about our books, find
us on Facebook at Summersdale Publishers, on Twitter at
@Summersdale and on Instagram at @summersdalebooks
and get in touch. We'd love to hear from you!

Thanks very much for buying this Summersdale book.

www.summersdale.com

Image credits
p38 – women talking © Mary Long/Shutterstock.com
pp.106, 107, 108, 109 – yoga poses
© Tond Van Graphcraft/Shutterstock.com;
p.110 – man listening to music © Nadya_Art/Shutterstock.com;
p.113 – man asleep © Glinskaja Olga/Shutterstock.com